Healthcare and Food

Francesco Bruno · Marta Bertolaso ·
Adriano Fabris
Editors

Healthcare and Food

Epistemology, Ethics and Law

palgrave
macmillan

Editors
Francesco Bruno
Department of Science and Technology for Sustainable Development and One Health
Campus Bio-Medico University of Rome
Rome, Italy

Marta Bertolaso
Department of Science and Technology for Sustainable Development and One Health
Campus Bio-Medico University of Rome
Rome, Italy

Adriano Fabris
Department of Civilizations and Forms of Knowledge
University of Pisa
Pisa, Italy

ISBN 978-981-95-5898-8 ISBN 978-981-95-5899-5 (eBook)
https://doi.org/10.1007/978-981-95-5899-5

This Palgrave Macmillan imprint is published by the registered company Springer Nature Singapore Pte Ltd.
The registered company address is: 152 Beach Road, #21-01/04 Gateway East, Singapore 189721, Singapore

Acknowledgements

This volume is part of the outputs of the project "Integral WELL-being for human flourishing: healthcare and food from an ethical and legal perspective (I-WELL)" funded by the European Union under the National Recovery and Resilience Plan (PNRR), Mission 4, Component 2, Investment 1.1 "Fund for the National Research Program and Projects of Significant National Interest (PRIN)" (Prot. no. P2022MFWB9, Sector ERC SH2, CUP C53D23009930001).

We would like to thank our colleagues Gianluca Brunori (Pisa University, Italy), Elena Dell'Agnese (University of Milano Bicocca, Italy), Manca Erzetič (New University and the Institute Nova Revija for the Humanities, Ljubljana, Slovenia), Michela Lazzeroni (Pisa University, Italy), Eleonora Sirsi (Pisa University, Italy), Alfredo Rocha de la Torre (Universidad Pedagógica y Tecnológica de Colombia, Tunya, Colombia), Luca Valera (Universidad de Valladolid, Spain) for stimulating discussions and constructive feedback. We would also like to acknowledge the collaboration of Pierluigi Barrotta, Roberto Gronda, Bryan Irias Alfaro, Sara Pautasso (Pisa University Research group), whose contributions enriched this project.

Francesco Bruno
Marta Bertolaso
Adriano Fabris

Introduction

Over the past 20 years, the need to conceive nutrition and food as relevant to integral well-being has become more pressing. Until now, the relation between nutrition and food has never been conceived as an interplay of levels of analysis. From an epistemological point of view, the hypothesis of this book is that it is possible to interpret food as a biodynamical interface in human-environment interactions. Food "works" as an intermediary interface between us and the environment but also between us and the social and cultural dimension. The fundamental idea of this book is a relational understanding of human beings. Considering that contextual and nutritional factors are relevant to understanding and treating complex diseases leads to the idea of a relational and systemic approach. This means that it cannot be ignored that human beings are relational entities that establish complex relationships with the environment and other human beings through the mediation of food. This approach links human flourishing with contextual factors, history, and the relational dimension. This new understanding of food as an interface is a requirement for developing a new ethical and legal framework which can effectively regulate the food chain in the future.

In this sense, an interdisciplinary approach is essential. Its main objective is to investigate the *epistemological*, *legal*, and *ethical* conditions that enable to achieve comprehensive well-being, both individually and collectively, from the perspective of nutritional health. In this sense, the aim is to develop a philosophical, ethical, and legal foundation of an integral well-being guided by food and nutrition, as a driver of change in order to promote a more sustainable future. Specifically, the aim is to demonstrate: (1) the positive role of a *relational epistemology*[1] and *ethics* in deepening the idea of food health; (2) the generative relationship between sustainability and integral well-being in practice (*ethics*); (3) the importance of best practices, codes of conduct and guidelines in reaching the goal of a more sustainable perspective on food health (*ethics and law*).

This book focuses on the development of "best practices," still not adequately addressed in ethical and legal fields. Thus, it intends to give a concrete contribution to the present challenges related not only to health but also, more broadly, to sustainable development and "food health," which is recognized as the relationship between well-being and nutrition. In order to achieve said goal, our proposal is to take into consideration both the notions of complexity and integrated development in light of a *systemic epistemology*, as well as the notions of nutrition, care, and health. Furthermore, this book focuses on some key aspects of the *communication* processes regarding food health within the *public sphere*, and the *ethical principles* underlying them. It delves into the relationship between experts and society, into the character of advertising and some controversial phenomena of social media food representation.

Such analysis will contribute to the elaboration of appropriate ethical elements that can promote an effective and correct food communication in the digital environments. Starting from this new approach, this book aims at the development and implementation of both ethical and legal codes of conduct for producers, restaurateurs, consumers, and communicators all over the food supply chain in order to promote the above mentioned integral well-being.

---

[1] In general, "relational epistemology" means that knowledge and definitions are strictly dependent on context. This approach allows the pluralism of reality to be safeguarded within the unity of knowledge (Bertolaso Marinucci 2024).

Starting from a relational epistemology, well-being and nutrition are not only inserted in an ethical-social context, but also in a legal context. Both regulate the relationships between human beings, food, and the environment. These relationships must obviously be sustainable. In fact, such sustainability is conventionally understood to entail the simultaneous pursuit of three main goals which are: environmental protection, social equity, and economic welfare. The Brundtland Commission of the UN defined sustainability and sustainable development as something that "meets the needs of the present without compromising the ability of future generations to meet their own needs"[2]. This definition brought the above mentioned terms into public debate. Sustainability involves a very wide range of interests which space from ethics and economics to environmental protection and also nutrition and food. Nutrition and food are recognized as the most highly contributing factors for integral well-being. For instance, under the 17 Sustainable Development Goals, "Not Hunger" is the second one which aims to "end hunger, achieve food security and improve nutrition and promote sustainable agriculture." This highlights a strong interplay between several sectors, such as agriculture, food security, nutrition, and food. These sentences raise the issue of a new relational perspective to conceive them in an original way. In this sense, "Not Hunger" appears to be more of a principle to strive toward than a real and effective goal. The situation can change by focusing attention on the concrete reality within a relational approach.

In the past twenty years, the need to safeguard consumers, public security, and the ecosystems has led to the development of new sets of rules. As a result, the concept of "Food health" has emerged (Bruno, 2017). Food health is recognized as the *relationship* between well-being and nutrition and is considered a key for human well-being. However, from an international legal point of view, there is still no shared corpus,

[2] See: https://www.are.admin.ch/are/en/home/media/publications/sustainable-development/brundtland-report.html

such as hard law, that can really have binding effects on food, environment, and health. If public and private behaviors are often oriented by the economy to the detriment of food and environmental health, a change is needed that also involves ethics and law, starting from the epistemological sphere.

For these reasons, the book aims to combine and integrate three fundamental aspects of nutrition.

Epistemology. Many different aspects are intertwined, from which emerges the need for an epistemological study. Applied science is often based on reductionist logics. These are not able to address and resolve the problems of an increasingly complex reality. Added to this need is the relational aspect typical of studies on the sustainability of the relationship between man and nature. Starting from an epistemology of complexity (Bertolaso & Marinucci 2024), new epistemological tools will be the basis for thinking about the relationship between nutrition, ethics, and law to preserve well-being and health.

Ethics. From an ethical perspective, well-being is a multidisciplinary relational concept, with different and distinctive meanings in several disciplines. It has a central role in ethics, medicine, psychology, economics, among others (Griffin, 1986; Fletcher, 2016a; Fletcher,. 2016b). The so-called Food ethics is the discipline that deals with such issues, highlighting their ethical dimension and identifying the key values and moral questions involved (Sandler 2015; Rawlinson & Ward, 2016; Barnhill et al., 2018). A more comprehensive approach to food ethics takes its bearings from the idea that every time we eat, we imply, promote, and establish relationships (Fabris, 2024). Starting from the idea that eating is a relational act, it is very important to offer a method that allows to place a given issue in the broader context of relations between health and environment (Fabris, 2019; Perullo, 2016).

Law. From a legal perspective, the right to food is "the right to have a regular, permanent and free access, either directly or by means of financial purchases, to quantitatively and qualitatively adequate and sufficient food corresponding to the cultural traditions of the people to which the consumer belongs, and which ensures a physical and mental, individual and collective, fulfilling and dignified life free of fear" (Ziegler, 2004). The problem is to highlight the inconsistencies between different jurisdictions, national and international (Bruno, 2017), and to propose general solutions. The relational approach allows us to reconcile different positions, without polarizing the general debate.

These issues structure the book as follows. The first part of the book intends to overcome the reductionist approach to nutrition, proposing a relational perspective. This allows us to conceive emerging phenomena as possibilities beyond the determination. It is about dealing with complexity and the resulting indeterminacy. Although it is not always possible to control a complex system, it is possible to manage it through an epistemology of uncertainty, which consists in providing a specific epistemological status to probability and uncertainty. The main concepts that will be explored are those of complex or non-linear causality, risk, probability, and uncertainty. The application of this new epistemology to the food sector allows to conceive food as a relational interface, which includes health, nutrition, and sustainability, especially where science does not provide certain answers to social, political, and legal issues.

The second part of the book will analyze some aspects of this food relationship. From an ethical perspective, the question is what determines an individual's well-being is a question that needs a comprehensive and multifaceted answer. Nutrition and food are two of these elements, as "Eating well" is certainly a part of well-being. But what does "well" mean in this case? This is an ethical concept that can only be addressed relationally and in an interdisciplinary manner. In this context, new lines of inquiry are emerging: food citizenship, i.e., reflection on the right of all human beings not to be just consumers at the end of the food chain, but participants in the food system as a whole; food security and food safety, i.e., research aimed at ensuring, on one hand, the safety of the food chain and, on the other, a correct relationship between food and health. Every activity related to food establishes and is a relationship. From this point of view, it is necessary to consider nutrition starting from the interactions that give it meaning and sense. The act of eating is relational since it involves the individuals in a relationship with food, with non-human animals, with the ecosystem, with other human beings, and with their cultures. The relational approach is, therefore, increasingly present both from a theoretical and ethical point of view. It is also present in Eastern tradition, as discussed in this book.

The third part of this book focuses on legal issues that have a significant social impact. From a legal point of view, Bruno (2017) shows that there is legislation on food, but there is no single legal corpus. This creates strong inhomogeneities in global food law between European and US law and the WTO. An integrated and relational approach reveals new possibilities for rethinking laws, as shown by the examples in this part of the book.

Francesco Bruno
Università Campus Bio-Medico di Roma
Marta Bertolaso
Università Campus Bio-Medico di Roma
Adriano Fabris
University of Pisa, Department of Civilisation and Forms of Knowledge

References

Barnhill, A., Budolfson, M., and Doggett, T., (2018) *The Oxford Handbook of Food Ethics*. Oxford University Press.
Bertolaso, M. & Marinucci, A. (2024). *Le questioni aperte della vita*. Rubbettino.
Bruno (2017). *Il diritto alimentare nel contesto globale: USA e UE a confronto*. Wolters Kluwer.
Fabris, A. (2019). *Etica del mangiare: cibo e relazione*. Edizioni ETS.
Fabris, A. (2024). *Ethics of Eating and Drinking*. Springer.
Fabris, A. (2024). *Ethics of Eating and Drinking*. Springer.
Fletcher, G. (2016a). *The philosophy of wellbeing. An Introduction*. Routledge.
Fletcher, G. (Ed.). (2106b). *The Routledge Handbook of wellbeing*. Routledge.
Griffin, J. (1986). *Wellbeing: its meaning, measurement and moral importance*. Clarendon Press.
Rawlinson, M. & Ward, C. (Eds). (2016). *The Routledge Handbook of Food Ethics*. Routledge.
Perullo, N. (2016). *Il gusto come esperienza: Saggio di filosofia ed estetica del cibo*. Slow Food Editore.
Sandler, R. (2015). *Food Ethics: The Basic*. Routledge.

Ziegler, J. (2004). *Special Rapporteur on the Right to Food, defended before the general Assembly in Nov. A/59/385, Para 5.* https://www.daccesiddsUn.org/doc/UNDoc/GEN/No4/525/17/PDF;.

Contents

Notes on Contributors

Marta Bertolaso is Full Professor of Philosophy of Science and Human Development at the University Campus Bio-Medico of Rome. Her expertise in philosophy of science, scientific practice and in philosophy of the life sciences has allowed her to promote and collaborate in interdisciplinary research and educational projects on complex and adaptive systems, and on human-environment interactions also when mediated by technology. The focus on the epistemological issues that emerge within the contemporary transitions has allowed her to contribute to normative and policy research programs too. Among other commitments, she is ordinary member of the "Académie Internationale de Philosophie des Sciences" and Editor in Chief of Springer Series on "Human Perspectives in Health Sciences and Technology".

Giacomo Brioni holds a Ph.D. in Philosophy from the Universities of Pisa and Florence. The main focus of his research is the relation between public choice theory, contractarianism, and political realism. He is also interested in the history of contemporary liberalism and in the thought of Leo Strauss.

Francesco Bruno is an attorney qualified for the Higher Courts and Full Professor at the Campus Bio-medical University of Rome (UCBM). He has been Visitor at Columbia Law School of New York (Center of Climate Change Law) in 2012, Visiting Faculty at UCLA School of Law in 2013 and 2014 and Visiting Researcher at Florida International University (FIU) in 2015. He is the author of over 100 scientific publications, books, papers, essays and articles. In Environmental and H&S Law, Francesco assists multinational companies and primary Italian companies with reference to criminal responsibility (environmental crimes and the safety of citizens and workers), administrative (sanctions, authorization procedures, relations with the public administration and appeals) and civil responsibility, providing legal assistance both in Court and by supporting Clients in the ordinary or extraordinary management of the company. In the field of Food Law, he has gained relevant experience regarding the entire food chain, relations with consumers and in all matters relating to product safety, under the various criminal, administrative and civil profiles. He is "probiviro" of "Federalimentare" since 2021 and a member of the National Food Safety Committee (CNSA) since 2022.

Ginevra Brutto is a Ph.D. student at the University Campus Bio-Medico of Rome with a research project entitled Nutraceuticals and the market between food regulations and pharmaceutical legislation: a reinterpretation of the rules governing production, marketing, and consumption and a Fellow of the Food Science and Human Nutrition Philosophy of Science research unit.

Sandra G. F. Bukkens is a researcher in the field of human nutrition and food systems. She worked at the Rowett Research Institute, Aberdeen, UK; Cornell University, Ithaca, NY, USA; the Italian National Research Institute for Food and Nutrition, Rome; the University of Padova, Italy; and the Institute of Environmental Science and Technology of the Universitat Autònoma de Barcelona, Spain. Currently she is affiliated with the European Centre for Governance in Complexity in Norway and the Universidad Científica del Sur in Peru. Her research has focused on energy metabolism, entomophagy, and multi-criteria evaluation of the performance of food systems in both developed and developing societies. In addition, she has vast experience in the management of European research projects and the organization of international conferences, workshops, and summer schools.

Camilla Clerici is an external consultant for the BRIC-Inail 2022 project "Protection of consumer workers in the food supply chain: regulatory aspects and preparation of specific policies in implementation of an integrated One Health approach" and has a Second Level Master's Degree in Food Law at LUISS Guido Carli University. Research fellow in 2020/2021 for the project "Project for the co-creation and regeneration of sustainable solutions with a high content of cultural, social, and institutional innovation" at the Department of Law of the University of Macerata, in the field of European food law and constitutional law.

Gelsomina Russo Corvace is a Ph.D. candidate and Research Fellow at Università Campus BioMedico di Roma with a project entitled "Sustainable development, climate change and the food enterprise: prospects for reforming European regulations". Her research activity is currently being conducted at the Faculty of Science and Technology for Sustainable Development and "One Health", Research Unit of Food Science and Nutrition.

Silvia Dadà is a tenure-track researcher in Moral Philosophy and Bioethics at the University of Pisa and she works on the PNRR FAIR project. Her research focuses on care ethics, bioethics, and AI ethics, especially vulnerability. She authored "Vulnerabilità digitale. Etica, Intelligenza Artificiale", Medicina (Mimesis, 2024).

Adriano Fabris is full professor of Moral Philosophy at the University of Pisa, where he also teaches Ethics of Communication. At the same University he is director of the Interdisciplinary Centre for Research in Communication. He is president of the National Society of Philosophy, Italy (Consulta Nazionale di Filosofia: https://www.consultanazionalef ilosofia.it), and a member of the Board of Directors of the Golinelli Foundation (https://www.fondazionegolinelli.it). He is currently co-PI of the Transversal Project on AI Ethics and Deontology of the PNRR Fair Project (https://future-airesearch.it/) and President (with Alfredo Rocha de la Torre) of the International Center of Studies on Contemporary Nihilism (based at the University of Tunja, Colombia: https://nihilismocontemporaneo.com.co). He is also director of the research Institute ReTe (Religions and Theology) of the University of Lugano (USI), Faculty of Theology, Switzerland (https://istitutorete.ch). On this field he promoted researches on inter-religious dialogue, on digital religions, and an international Master degree online on "Science, Philosophy and Theology of Religions". Among his recent publications: Ethics of Information and Communication Technology (Springer, Cham 2018); Trust. A Philosophical Approach (ed., Springer, Cham 2020); Ethics of Eating and Drinking. Food and Relations (Springer, Cham 2024); Digital Environments and Human Relations (ed. with S. Belardinelli, Springer, Cham 2024).

Mario Giampietro recently retired from the Catalan Institution for Research and Advanced Studies (ICREA), Barcelona. Until September 2023, he was ICREA Research Professor at the Institute of Environmental Science and Technology of the Universitat Autònoma de Barcelona, Spain, where he dedicated his academic career to the integrated assessment of (uncomfortable) sustainability issues using concepts from complex systems theory. Presently he is collaborating with the European Centre for Governance in Complexity (ECGC) in Norway, where his research is focused on the bioeconomy, biosemiotics, and governance in complexity. He has (co)authored over 150 publications, including six books. ICREA: https://www.icrea.cat/Web/ScientificStaff/Mario-giampietro-423

Seung Chul Kim, born in Seoul, Korea, in 1958. Awarded Dr. theol. at the Faculty of Theology of the University of Basel in 1989. Since 2012, he has been a permanent research fellow at the Nanzan Institute for Religion and Culture at Nanzan University in Japan. His research includes the themes of interreligious dialogue, Bioethics, and religious literature.

Jacopo Marchetti is a Postdoctoral Researcher at the University of Pisa, where he teaches Political Communication and earned his Ph.D. in Political Philosophy in 2019. He authored *Foucault e Hayek. Tra biopolitica e liberalismo* (IBL, 2018) and *Douglass C. North* (IBL, 2021), and he edited *Il potere della menzogna. Comunicazione e politica nella società digitale* (Il Mulino, 2024).

Angelo Marinucci is a researcher at the Campus Bio-Medico University in Rome. His research interests include epistemology, theoretical biology and physics. His main publications include "Theoretical Principles of Relational Biology" (Springer 2023).

Antonio Masala is Associate Professor of Political Philosophy at the Department of Civilisations and Forms of Knowledge, University of Pisa. His research interests include classical liberal political philosophy, populism, and the social and political impact of artificial intelligence.

Veronica Neri is Associate Professor of Moral Philosophy at the University of Pisa, where she teaches Media Ethics. She is a member of the Ph.D. Program Board in Philosophy at the Universities of Pisa and Florence, and serves on the editorial board of the journal "Teoria". Her latest publications include contributions on the ethics of public communication, advertising and fashion ethics, media ethics, and the ethical implications of visual media and artificial intelligence, published in both national and international journals.

Roger Strand is Professor at the Centre for the Study of the Sciences and the Humanities at the University of Bergen (Norway), as well as Co-Director of the European Centre for Governance in Complexity. His research focuses on uncertainty and complexity at the interfaces between science and institutions of governance.

List of Figures

The Complexity of Food Health Related Choices

Epistemology and Sciences

The Epistemological Status of Uncertainty and the Precautionary Principle

Angelo Marinucci and Marta Bertolaso

1 Introduction

The eighteenth-and nineteenth-century (and partly contemporary) hope of a science capable of revealing all the secrets of nature through mathematics able to show its essence, are shattered 1 by the "negative" result of Poincaré (three-body problem) (Barrow-Green, 1997) that opened the way to deterministic chaos in physics (Marinucci, 2011) and 2 by the complexity of the biological systems (Bertolaso & Marinucci, 2024).

There are phenomena that are perfectly predictable, in which it is possible to identify the causes, the effects and their interactions in a completely explicit and deterministic way. Cases of this type allow for almost total predictability and control. These safe islands are surrounded by oceans in which the complexity of the systems reduces control and

A. Marinucci (✉) · M. Bertolaso
Università Campus Bio-Medico di Roma, Rome, Italy
e-mail: angelico937@gmail.com

M. Bertolaso
e-mail: m.bertolaso@unicampus.it

F. Bruno et al. (eds.), *Healthcare and Food*,
https://doi.org/10.1007/978-981-95-5899-5_1

predictability to the point of making them impossible. For this reason, it was necessary to develop methods and theories to manage complexity, without the pretension of solving it. Many of these are linked to how knowledge is developed and interpreted. If scientists do not work on dry land, it is nevertheless possible to navigate the ocean of complexity, with due care.

Nowadays, science is generally well aware of its condition, however it is not always perceived in this way. In society, politics and jurisprudence, the idea that science is always able to provide solid and incontrovertible certainties is in fact usually consolidated (Benessia et al. 2016). For this reason, on scientific issues which have political, legal and social value (such as nutrition, health, environment, sustainability) politics and justice decide and choose starting from scientific advice in the firm belief of always receiving incontrovertibly certain answers. This belief is not based on scientific thinking, but on technological thinking that thinks starting from optimizations.

In this regard, this text analyzes the precautionary principle (Section 4), both as an example of what is being said and to try to apply to it an epistemology of uncertainty, new to the political and legal fields. However, it is necessary to begin with a detailed and epistemological discussion of the theoretical bases that allow us to think about complexity, indeterminacies and the new challenges of knowledge. They also concern the political, administrative and legal fields. First of all, it is necessary to understand how to think about an epistemology of certainty (Section 2) and one of uncertainty (Section 3).

As said, the actual existence of completely predictable phenomena does not exhaust all of reality, rather it constitutes a minimal part of it. For this reason, it is necessary to dwell on these two epistemologies, and then apply them to the precautionary principle, which will allow introducing a new epistemology within the legal and political spheres. It is fundamentally a question of conceiving in a new way the relationship between the object of knowledge and the real object, the general approach to knowledge and some aspects of the concept of cause between determinism and complexity.

2 Epistemology of Certainty

The topic of the epistemology of certainty will be treated in such a way as to highlight the points that, on the one hand, have allowed the resolution of many questions and an important progress in knowledge, on the other hand, have left out of knowledge everything to which "certainty" cannot be applied. It is true that each method illuminates a specific area of reality, however the problem is that the area in which uncertainty prevails is much wider.

Only recently, between the end of the nineteenth century and the beginning of the twentieth century, and especially since the end of the 1960s, scientists have dealt with complex phenomena, that is, with what cannot be reduced to the sum of its elements. Today, complexity is used not only in science, but also in the social sciences, in business management, in politics, etc. If one wants to get to the heart of the matter, it is necessary to recognize that Laplace and Poincaré have delimited the scientific and philosophical terms of this question. It is worth quoting them because they are extremely clear and because they are more than current.

Much of the question about the proximities and, above all, about the differences between epistemology of certainty and epistemology of uncertainty is summarized in two quotes from the two scientists just mentioned.

> We ought to regard the present state of the universe as the effect of its antecedent state and as the cause of the state that is to follow. An intelligence knowing all the forces acting in nature at a given instant, as well as the momentary positions of all things in the universe, would be able to comprehend in one single formula the motions of the largest bodies as well as the lightest atoms in the world, provided that its intellect were sufficiently powerful to subject all data to analysis; to it nothing would be uncertain, the future as well as the past would be present to its eyes (Laplace 1967, p. 243).

> If we knew exactly the laws of nature and the state of the universe at the initial instant, we could predict what the state of this same universe would

> be at a subsequent instant. But even if the laws of nature no longer had any secrets for us, we could only know the initial state approximately. If this allows us to know the subsequent state with the same approximation, we need nothing else, and we will say that the phenomenon has been predicted, that there are laws that govern it. But this is not always the case: it can happen that small differences in the initial conditions generate very large differences in the final phenomena; a small error regarding the former would then generate an enormous error regarding the latter. Prediction becomes impossible, we are faced with a fortuitous phenomenon (Poincaré 2006, pp. 107–108).

The first quote from Laplace is less and less known today, while it is really difficult to find quotes from the second. This is partially also due to the wide literature in the complexity science of the last century (e.g., Weaver 1948, Wimsatt 2007, Mitchell 2009, Bertolaso 2013b; Dupré and Nicholson 2018); however from a historical and didactic point of view, it is useful to follow the above-mentioned quotes and how they were related. In the first, a very close connection between determinism, causality and reductionism is implicit. From an intertextual point of view, it is immediately clear that Poincaré explicitly takes up Laplace's text, but makes small and crucial changes. Poincaré wants to place himself in the scientific tradition of Laplace and, at the same time, take a decisive step forward, creating a new field of investigation: deterministic chaos (Barrow-Green, 1997). Therefore, the entire previous scientific and epistemological tradition is expressed through Poincaré, precisely at the moment in which it distances itself, creating a new line of research.

In other words, Poincaré illuminates for the first time that broad area of reality in which it is not possible to determine and predict natural phenomena.

To understand what epistemologically changes, it is necessary to briefly dwell on deterministic epistemology because it is what is eventually present in technology and in the perception of science in politics and jurisprudence. Although the concepts used by Laplace today are rewritten, updated and clarified, nothing changes. What really changes are the approaches linked to the innovations introduced by Poincaré (Bocchi & Ceruti, 2007; Cini, 1999).

Determinism, Causality and Reductionism

It Is Important to Underline that Determinism, Causality and Reductionism Are the Key Concepts, whose Relationships Have Built a World and an Imaginary of Certainties in Science that Still Lasts Today. In the Previous Quote, Laplace States that if it Were Possible to Know Exactly the Initial Conditions of a Phenomenon, it Would Be Possible to Completely Predict the Future and Reconstruct the Past

This apparently simple statement hides many assumptions. First of all, it supports a substantial determinism. He states the existence of a bidirectional implication between determinism and predictability (determinism $\Leftrightarrow$ predictability) (Marinucci, 2011): if all the elements of a system are known, it is possible to predict all its configurations and vice versa. Furthermore, this implies the idea that it is possible to explain phenomena by reducing them to their simple elements. Reductionism is an extremely important concept because it has informed physics and biology. It is a concept that implies a specific ontology, because it claims to say something about how the world is structured. In this theoretical context, an ontological statement constitutes both reality and the way of knowing it. In this sense, non-deterministic forms of scientific knowledge (for example, probability) do not have an epistemological status of their own and are thought of as a distance from the truth.

For all this to be possible, Laplace presupposes that a direct proportionality is always maintained between causes and effects, so that the effect of a small perturbation can never determine the trajectory of an object and it will remain small.

> Most of the time, natural phenomena are complicated by extraneous causes: an enormous number of disturbing causes mix their influence, so much so that it is very difficult to recognize them. To achieve this, it is necessary to multiply observations or experiments, so that, by mutually destroying the extraneous effects, the average results highlight the phenomena and their various elements (Laplace, 1967, pp. 298–299).

This specific relationship between cause and effect, apparently banal, is extremely important because it is the element that Poincaré criticizes to open the way to dynamic systems and complexity. Furthermore, it is important because it represents the basis of a deterministic and completely controllable representation of the world. Linear causality (Bertolaso 2013a; Ilardo & Bertolaso, 2024) is precisely what binds events in an indissoluble way also in risk assessments and evaluations. With hindsight it is easy to affirm that not only causality or only this type of causality exists. However, it is necessary to underline this aspect because it is precisely the element on which the vulgate is based according to which science is considered able to always provide certain answers, precisely deterministic and causally characterizable. In fact, the clear and rigid physical distinction between causes and perturbations has its philosophical counterpart in the idea according to which it is always possible to distinguish the essential elements of a system from the accidental ones. From this point of view, the elements of a system are conceived as distinct and separate (Deleuze, 2004). The complete and well-formed definition of the individual elements of a system is generally the starting point of any epistemological or scientific investigation, within the epistemology of certainty. In this conceptual framework, the definition of distinct and separate elements is always the first step. Only subsequently do they interact. In this way, the interaction between the elements will produce effects that are completely predictable a priori. From the point of view of relationality and integration between the elements of a system, the consequence of this situation is that possibilities beyond determination are not conceivable, that is, it is hard to think of properties of a system that are not reducible to one another or the sum of its parts.

It is important to emphasize that this method is able to describe a part of the world; problems arise when it is considered ontologically, when a methodology becomes an ontology (Bertolaso, 2013b; Bertolaso & Kovacic, 2024), i.e., a statement about the world. From this point of view, the distinction between the object of knowledge and the real object is lost. If these coincide, reality is reduced to the perspective from which it is looked at. The presupposition of this approach to knowledge is Platonic, and it has been reinforced by the modern and Descartes naturalism and empiricisms. It consists in thinking that to describe how a phenomenon is, it is first necessary to say what it is and/or what its parts are, that is, it is necessary to define them. "To define" means to trace the boundaries of something (Wittgenstein 1999b). In this case, a definition becomes the conceptual boundary of something. In the analytical philosophy, this occurs by reducing objects to their constituent elements, again, by mereologically defining them.[1]

A clear example, in which the epistemology of certainty works is that of a car motor. Indeed, the functioning of the motor can be explained in a reductionistic and deterministic way, through a linear causality (Ilardo & Bertolaso, 2024). The elements of this system are really distinct and separate, defined before the interaction and are, subsequently, assembled (interaction) to obtain an effect analytically predicted a priori. Furthermore, in cases like this, the elements of an object or a system are defined first and then the context is considered. In reality, it will be seen that the context co-constitutes itself with the object of scientific investigation (Bailly e Longo, 2006). An analytical and reductionistic approach, based on the priority of the complete and well-formed definition, fails to grasp the intrinsic relationality, the co-constitution of object and context and their mutual co-implication because it considers them distinct and separate.

At the root of this philosophical-scientific framework, there is a specific interpretation of nonlinear differential equations. From a physical point of view, between the eighteenth and twentieth centuries these were considered as a linear equation plus one or more perturbations. As mentioned above, it is not trivial to remember that scientists before Poincaré thought that perturbations always had negligible effects on physical dynamics (*cause and effect are directly proportional*[2]).

Specifically, being able to solve physical problems meant, in the context of modern physics, having to deal with linear mathematical problems, or in any case being able to reduce everything to them, as they were considered problems not only solvable mathematically, but their solubility was guaranteed by nature itself (Marinucci, 2011).

[1] In Section 3, the epistemology of uncertainty will be introduced. It is a different approach that allows us to describe cases in which science does not provide certainty as in life.

[2] Interesting historical examples of this question are: (Euler, 1960a, Euler, 1960b).

The linearity of a differential equation, as well as the possible linearization, was the mathematical element of the presumption of being able to know the past and the future globally, since the mathematical evolution of the dynamics could be followed and predicted without having to deal with the sensitivity to the initial conditions (Israel, 1991). Linearity was the fulcrum around which the possibility of answering the question of certain knowledge was gathered. From this perspective, "linearizing" did not only mean making a nonlinear equation tractable, but it meant, more precisely, discovering the linear term, responsible for the overall trend of a dynamics. From this point of view, every complex problem becomes complicated and, therefore, solvable analytically through the identification of its simple components.

The Concept of Combinatorial Interaction

One of the Elements on which it Is Essential to Focus Attention, to Better Understand What Has Been Said, Is the Methodological-Philosophical Approach of Analytical Reductionism. It Is Necessary to Summarize it Briefly because it Allows us to Clarify how to Understand the Concept of Interaction, which Is Fundamental in Complex Systems. In this Sense, it Is Necessary to Properly Distinguish between "Reductionism" and "Reduction." the Latter Is a Fundamental Scientific Practice that Has Allowed Achieving Numerous Results, as Shown, for Example, by Eighteenth-Century Science. It Consists in Breaking down a Problem, So as to Be Able to Look for the Simple Elements through which to Describe it. Therefore, Reduction Has an Ineliminable Heuristic Value

On the contrary, reductionism is not an activity, but a philosophical concept. It consists in thinking that solving a problem in general means breaking it down[3] to reach its constituent elements. Once isolated, these are able to offer a complete picture of what we intend to know (Descartes, 2000).

Unlike reduction, reductionism has an epistemological value, to which it is possible to associate, as has been done, an ontological meaning, such

[3] For this reason, it is necessary to speak of analytical reductionism.

that through analytical reductionism it would become possible to reveal the secrets of nature.

Now, the scientific practice of reducing a phenomenon to its constituent elements does not immediately imply philosophical positions on knowledge in general: selecting elements does not necessarily mean identifying the essence of something, but it can mean choosing elements that are relevant for a description of a phenomenon.

Despite this important difference, reduction and reductionism have assumed a semantic field not far apart in the history of science. Scientific practice was (and often is) conceived within a fundamental reductionism. It imposed itself thanks to the successes of physics and was structured around ontological and epistemological assumptions, for which knowing was synonymous with grasping the essence.

As mentioned, within a reductionist methodology, knowing means isolating and defining the constituent elements of a system, to which it will be possible to reduce all the properties and, more generally, everything that concerns the interaction of the same first elements.

In this way, a conceptual space is delimited within which the possible configurations of a system are found. The consequence is that the end and the purpose of the solution of a problem coincides with the delimitation of its conceptual space, whose simple elements are able to clarify it in all its parts. In this sense, from time to time, a configuration of a phenomenon will present itself in reality, which can only be a concretization of one of the possibilities which are analytically determined a priori.

In short, we call "combinatorial interaction" the philosophical idea according to which knowing something means isolating, abstracting and analytically defining its simple elements, such as to delimit a closed space in which the real object is completely predeterminable and controllable. In this case, the interaction between elements of a system and the system itself is conceived only and exclusively starting from their constituent elements.

Object of Knowledge and Real Object

If Epistemological and Ontological Values Are Associated with Combinatorial Interaction, a Method Becomes Not Only an Ontology but Also Imposes a Rationality. In Other Words, a Cognitive Tool Becomes the Way to Identify the Ultimate Nature of the Scientific Object. In this Sense, Delimiting a Closed Space Does Not Only Mean Solving a Problem, but Having a Criterion for Recognizing the Object as Susceptible to Scientific Treatment.

Dwelling on such an ontological and epistemological value means grasping its philosophical constraints, as profound as they are often invisible. By assuming that nature, or more generally a real object, has a certain type of rationality, it is bound to a single fundamental knowledge. In this way, it is no longer possible to admit the possibility of other methods,[4] since even the latter is bound within a mechanical and procedural rationality, so that knowing means rigorously following well-defined steps in order to reach the pre-established goal (Descartes, 2000). In other words, it is a matter of analytically identifying elements that can allow a complete and objective determination of the object. It is a matter of trying to define simple elements in order to be able to recognize what should be at that point considered the real object as an object of knowledge as such, even before actually knowing it.

The presence of strong epistemological and, above all, ontological assumptions about nature and knowledge essentially imposes two constraints, one formal and one content-related. The first refers to the recognizability of the real object and the constitution of the object of knowledge; the second concerns the fact that once the essential elements of something are identified and delimited, these do not change, precisely because they assume an ontological status.

Hence, knowing something means rigidly delimiting a conceptual space, on the basis of which essential and accidental elements of a phenomenon are distinguished. A complete and well-formed definition

[4] In this context, the possibility of other methods cannot but be something qualitatively inferior to the method that captures its essence. For example, an aesthetic description of the cosmos will certainly have less value than a mathematical and/or physical one.

is thus possible. In this case, precisely because of the ontological value, the object of knowledge and the real one coincide.

Consequently, only that for which an ontological space can be delimited can be the object of true and certain knowledge.

In such a structured conceptual space, what is outside the epistemological framework of the two constraints mentioned falls within the field of uncertainty. In this epistemological framework, uncertainty and probability do not have their own cognitive status. Therefore, they are thought of only as the measure of distance from the truth.[5] The aforementioned constraints impose that what can be known has to be characterized as stated. Everything to which such a rationality is not applicable is either something contingent or something for which it has not yet been possible to delimit a space of knowledge. At this point, the exclusivity of a rationality with ontological consequences and the consequent limits in which the description of reality is forced are evident.

As stated, where a conceptual space is defined, it can be considered complete and ontologically characterized. Consequently, it can only contain the essential elements able of fully and objectively explaining a phenomenon. In this way, all the possibilities of an object thus defined are found analytically in the essential elements that compose it.

In summary, if it is possible to think of an object by reducing it to its simplest and most essential elements through combinatorial interaction, then it is possible to know completely a priori all the possibilities of such an object. As we will see, what has been said is valid only within the limits of the elements identified. Considering this limitation, "object of knowledge" and "real object" do not coincide, the "object of knowledge" captures a particular aspect of the "real object."

[5] In the last part of this chapter, the debate on the precautionary principle will be introduced. In its formulations, this assumption is clearly perceived, that is, that decisions are made only starting from the certain answers of science. When this does not happen, provisional decisions are made, waiting for certainties, without considering that sometimes science cannot provide them. The same thing happened in the mid-eighteenth century during a smallpox epidemic (Paty, 1988). The problem was whether to inoculate it or not. D'Alembert thought that an uncertain tool such as probability could not be used to make this type of decision. In both cases, probability and everything that is uncertain do not have its own epistemological status. However, there are cases in which it is structurally not possible to go beyond this type of knowledge.

Reductionist and analytical approaches associate knowledge with an ontological value, so that the elements identified constitute its essence. Consequently, such a coincidence becomes the point at which the research on such a real object ends.

Therefore, the fact that an epistemological value is associated with combinatorial interaction allows it to become the rationality of nature. Consequently, knowing means applying this method to the purpose of the coincidence of the object of knowledge and the real object: here its ontological value is shown.

In this way, the fundamental properties of the object will be those analytically reducible to its simple elements. Consequently, the possibility is completely predetermined and immutable, within the space of possibilities constituted by combinatorial interaction. The ontological status is shown in the constraint whereby nothing else, outside of the simple elements, can account for a real object, and therefore modify its possibilities. In this sense, is it the same/very? field of (real) objectivity that is constituted and reduced to that of knowledge. It is characterized as the space by which and in which it is possible to recognize the scientific object. For example, for a certain period scientists called the "non-coded" parts of DNA "junk DNA" (Wells, 2011): they were not recognized as scientific objects of biological theory. Only that which is coded had an epistemological and ontological status. In this case, the identity between the object of knowledge and the real object is expressed in the identity between the metaphor of the code and DNA (and life), precisely reduced to code.

If the real object presents itself in a tangle of essential and accidental elements, knowing it means separating them through clear conceptual boundaries. In this way, the space of essence presents itself as something in which only one jurisdiction applies, in which all aspects of the object can be freed from the initial tangle. Thus they become completely determinable a priori, and in the same terms/through the same mereological categories.

In this perspective, the field of objectivity will be such as to admit only those possibilities that allow complete, objective and universal knowledge. In this methodological context, every single concept (knowledge) will always be identical to itself. In fact, it exhausts the possibilities of the real object a priori. As we will discuss more extensively in the following sections, the possibility to conceive the intrinsic dynamism of life and its complexity is lost (Bertolaso & Marinucci, 2024).

When the "object of knowledge" and the "real object" coincide, completeness, objectivity, timelessness and universality, which characterize the object of the (scientific) knowledge, determine whether it is possible to have scientific knowledge of a real object. If this is possible, a reductionist ontology is constituted.

However, the history of philosophy, the history of science, etc. show that as knowledge, social needs and cognitive tools change, and that certainties considered absolute can be strengthened or crumbled. Consequently, from the content point of view, it is necessary to at least weaken the scope of knowledge and its tools. In other words, this means weakening or not considering the content constraint.

In this way, it is necessary to introduce time, change, dynamism and history into knowledge, in order to question the exclusivity and static nature of the deterministic description of nature. More generally, the most important issue is to question the fact, not at all obvious, that knowing means knowing the essence. Inserting history into knowledge can be done in many ways. In the context of analytical reductionism, history enters into knowledge in a very specific sense: identifying the ways in which, from time to time, the object of knowledge has determined the real one, characterizing it differently over time.

In this sense, by inserting time, only the epistemological and ontological status of the content of knowledge is called into question, but not its form. History can thus appear only and exclusively as a succession of closed definitions, just like those that need to be questioned. Admitting, therefore, that knowledge differs within different moments or contexts, does not necessarily mean thinking differently. We will expand on this in the following section.

Within the philosophical debate on the legal principle of precaution, there is a great discussion on the need for a complete and universal definition of precaution. Different definitions of precaution have been proposed because it would be necessary to look for a definition, that is, to delimit and close the conceptual space of precaution. In this sense, it will be important to argue that it is more important to focus on the theoretical role of a "principle" than on a complete and objective definition of precaution. The discussion between the various definitions of precaution is fundamental, but it is always found within the same philosophical analytical context.

Conceiving the historicity of knowledge as a progress toward something like truth (even if only teleologically reachable), precisely what was intended to be overcome returns. In other words, it becomes impossible to escape from an epistemology that, by constraining the form of knowledge, remains in a particular space of constitution of the object. This has a methodological value, since it certainly admits more contents (for example more definitions of precaution), but all constituted in the same way.

On the contrary, it is necessary to question the very constitution of the scientific object, that is, of the formal constraint. It is now possible to understand what it means that Poincaré managed to open up a new part of the world. The crucial point is, in fact, the escape from the formal constraint that restrains knowledge.

From this perspective, the concept of combinatorial interaction, understood as an approach and method, offers concrete and fertile ground for proposing and discussing something different.

In summary, the theoretical option discussed so far can explain phenomena either by reducing them to their simple elements or by constituting a closed conceptual space whose possible configurations are known a priori. Within this space it is possible to conceive and predict the evolution of a phenomenon. From the point of view of knowledge, there are constraints that constitute the scientific "object of knowledge" and that allow recognizing the "real object" as susceptible to scientific knowledge. These are the formal constraint and the content constraint. This is based on the ontological and epistemological status of reductionism. Furthermore, the brief discussion of historicity in this epistemology does not change the way of knowing.

3 Epistemology of Uncertainty

If it is not possible to predetermine the configurations of a phenomenon through a reductionist and analytical method, the problem becomes to conceive possibilities beyond determination. In other words, these are possibilities that, although they are not determinable, have at least to be conceivable, in order to be able to manage them. This is fundamental to be able to decide in situations of uncertainty, in the medical, political, legal, environmental fields, etc.

Epistemology and Complexity

As Regards the Double Implication Determinism $\Leftrightarrow$ Predictability, Poincaré Is in Continuity with Laplace because Predictability $\Rightarrow$ Determinism Remains Valid, but he Distances himself because it Is Not Always True that Knowing Everything about a System, it Is Possible to Predict all its Configurations. From Here, after Poincaré Determinism $\nRightarrow$ Predictability Becomes a New Possibility because there Really Are Systems in which Determinism $\Rightarrow$ Predictability[6] (Marinucci, 2011). Already in Poincaré's Time, and Especially Today, there Was the Problem of Managing Situations of Uncertainty. These Are Due to the Indeterminability of Many Complex Phenomena.

In nature there are many types of complex phenomena, linked to different fields of research: physics, biology, social sciences, etc. If I said that in exactly one year in Rome it will be sunny, many would say that the prediction is absurd and that if I guessed it would be by pure chance. On the contrary, if I said that in exactly one year the earth will be more or less in the same position with respect to the sun, no one would have anything to object. From a mathematical point of view, these are two phenomena described by nonlinear differential equations that cannot be integrated and are globally unstable. The difference is that in the first

[6] From a mathematical point of view, generally the most frequent type of differential equations are the non-linear non-integrable ones. After Poincaré, reductionism, determinism and linear causality enter into crisis because these concepts are not always able to explain complex phenomena.

case the reliability of the prediction is very low, in the second it is very high. There is no need to dwell on the mathematical details,[7] but it is possible to calculate the reliability of the prediction of phenomena such as the previous ones. These examples show that, although it is not possible to control certain phenomena, it is possible to manage them and conceive possible configurations through scientific tools. However, these do not provide any definitive answer on the possible and real states of the system.

The answers remain open, the concepts remain undefined, but they can be defined in the particularity of a context. It is precisely here that the difference between managing and controlling a phenomenon emerges clearly. As seen, weather forecasts are reliable for a few hours, but they are never certain. From this perspective, it is possible to define something by delimiting a context and/or an interface (Arora et al., 2020) through which it is analyzed. The same can be said of the solar system: the reliability of forecasts is enormous, but it is limited. At this point, a fundamental uncertainty emerges that imposes itself. Nonetheless, it is possible to make decisions starting from the lack of certainty.

Precisely this uncertainty has to be thought of in order to make it manageable, as much as possible. It is certainly possible to know something, to provide an answer, but this does not mean dominating reality, but rather managing it. Managing means being able to make decisions on uncertainties, governing (Bertolaso & Kovacic, 2024) concrete problems. It is an uncertainty that is part of everyday life.[8]

In the life sciences, the situation becomes much more complicated. Biological generalizations and abstractions have a specific characteristic. For example, by abstracting from the study of multiple phenotypes of the same species, it is always possible to observe general properties. However, these do not have an ontological status because the singularity of living beings (Bailly & Longo, 2006) is sacrificed. Generalizations and abstractions are very useful tools for talking about a group of individuals. "Species," "family," etc. serve precisely this purpose, but individuals

---

[7] On the mathematical details, see (Tabor, 1989).

[8] From a scientific point of view, almost all of the equations that describe physical and biological reality are nonlinear and non-integrable: Poincaré really illuminated an enormous space.

of a species always maintain their own singularity (Bailly & Longo, 2006, Darwin, 1859). It is undoubtedly possible to talk about groups of individuals (species) and manage problems related to them. However, biological generalizations do not capture the differences that constitute individuals despite their similarity. This aspect emerged clearly during the last pandemic, considering the effects of vaccinations and the virus on individuals.

Considering what has been said, the object of knowledge and the real object no longer coincide. The instrument of knowledge does not faithfully reflect nature, but it is something that is applied to nature (Kant, 1996). In fact, nature answers our questions: the instruments of knowledge illuminate aspects of nature, in the sense that they allow us to manage phenomena, even when there are no certainties. The examples proposed show well that it is necessary to describe how a system is and what configuration it has assumed to say what it is, to define an aspect in a context.

As regards causality, it has been seen that it is not necessary to maintain a direct proportionality between causes and effects. Therefore, if a small cause can have a determining effect on a phenomenon, it is necessary to activate the system to understand what configuration it will have. From this point of view, causality acts in a complex manner. The elements of a system act together, co-determining each other and giving rise to something irreducible. In the next paragraph, it will be seen that they are no longer primarily distinct and separate, but can be conceived as distinct and inseparable.[9]

When dealing with complexity and emergent phenomena, it is precisely something that cannot be reduced to its constituent elements. This last characterization is only negative; talking about "indeterminability" is not enough. It is necessary to fill the conceptual space that opens up, toward an epistemology of complexity (Bertolaso & Marinucci, 2024). It forms the backdrop to an epistemology of uncertainty.[10] In this way, an epistemological status can be given to the tools that allow

[9] This distinction is found in (Deleuze, 2004). It is reworked and applied to complexity.

[10] In addition to its usefulness in science, this approach can also be used profitably in other areas. In this regard, the precautionary legal principle will be explored in the last part of this chapter.

managing uncertainty. This enables and legitimates to make decisions in all areas where uncertainties arise (not only related to science) such as medicine, politics and law.

The Concept of Relation

If the Concept of Combinatorial Interaction Is Necessary and Useful to Explain a Series of Phenomena, it cannot Be Extended to any Phenomenon. It Is Limiting in the Scientific Practices of Analysis of Reality, both for Scientific and Social Use. As Seen, Combinatorial Interaction Implies the Idea that Reality Is Controllable and Predictable through Science. As Mentioned, it Presupposes and Is Structured on Specific Constraints. These Are Particularly Important because they Allow us to Conceive an Epistemology of Complexity, Once Questioned

It has been said that it is not always possible to predict all the configurations of a complex system. From this point of view, it is necessary to "activate" the system to see which configurations it assumes. For this reason, it is necessary to reverse the fundamental philosophical questions: the description of a phenomenon (how) allows us to define it (what) from time to time (Wittgenstein, 1999a; Wittgenstein, 1999b). This simple change in the way of thinking has profound consequences capable of positively characterizing the world of complexity.

If it is not possible to define a phenomenon with certainty and completeness, this does not prevent it from being treated differently. Poincaré's quote shows that it is not necessary to maintain proportionality between causes and effects. An apparently irrelevant cause can have determining effects on the dynamics to be described. If therefore the configuration that a phenomenon will take is not predictable, it is first necessary to describe how to define it. In other words, the description (how) of the phenomenon allows it to be defined, to say what it is.

In this case, building a definition presupposes the choice of a level of description, that is, an interface that literally allows you to see the phenomenon or the emergent property. Choosing, for example, a level that is too low, such as that of the elements of the system, does not allow access to the emergent properties to be described.[11] Knowledge becomes irremediably complex[12] and presents itself as relationally structured.[13] As regards different phenomena or single phenomena, several ways of questioning it are possible. Furthermore, different criteria may apply in different cases. For this reason, each time, depending on the questions that are asked, it will be a question of identifying what is most "pertinent" (Stengers, 2007) to solve the problem. From this point of view, the concept of interface is fundamental because it unites a particular perspective and its context of scientific investigation, as well as remaining open to a multiplicity of points of view.

A paradigmatic example of an interface can be a tissue compared to cancer cells. Cancer appears at the tissue level, even if it implies elements of a lower level (cell) and a higher level (organs). The tissue, in this case, sets the relationships from which cancer emerges. In this case, neoplastic cells appear as a consequence of the disruption of the inter-relations that hold the functional structure of the tissues itself. Moreover, tumor cells are actually identified, defined and inquired on the basis of their genealogical, functional and contextual life history. The very definition of tumor cell is therefore relational. In other terms, it is not possible to reconstruct a biological system or observable without taking into account the historicity of the organism, like in the case of cancer, form an epistemological point of view (Bertolaso, 2016; Bertolaso, 2013a). As a consequence, knowledge is always local, as it refers to a particular relational space. From a methodological point of view, it is a question of choosing a strategy suitable for the individual scientific question, not a universal method (Morin, 2007).

In a no-reductionist or systemic perspective, considering combinatorial and relational interaction, two qualitative descriptions of a phenomenon can be given in the first place. In the former, it is reduced

---

[11] There are many examples of emergent properties. Probably the simplest is represented by living beings in all their forms: it is not possible to conceive them starting from their simple elements or from their sum.

[12] This new perspective is even more interesting because it is able to include combinatorial interaction in itself. In fact, it can be considered as a level of description that allows access to some properties of the object. Some of these aspects are mentioned in (Morin, 2007).

[13] Combinatorial interaction can be thought of as a special case of relation. It is the relation in which the elements of a system can be considered as distinct and separate.

to simpler elements, while in the latter it is described as complex. However, the latter contains a plurality of perspectives. Concretely, there are approaches that illuminate different aspects of a phenomenon. For this reason, the more perspectives one has on a phenomenon, the more its effective knowledge increases.

If combinatorial interactions presuppose that the elements of a system are distinct and separate, in a perspective that is based on the relation, this characterization is not sufficient and not even epistemologically adequate.

In addition to the phenomena that can be explained by applying an epistemology of certainty, there is a complex part of the world that can be described and explained in a contextual and relational way. An epistemology that values uncertainty, giving it an epistemological status, is exactly what allows us to manage these situations. It is not always possible to abstract the object from its context in order to analytically derive the entire spectrum of possibilities that characterize it. If the possibility refers to a concrete space, then it is always possible to give an explanation, linked to a level of relevance, relative to an interface that provides access to the object of investigation.

Deleuze, states that "Descartes' error, which can be found in various texts, is that of having believed that the real distinction between parts implied their separability. [...]. According to Leibniz, however, two parts of matter that are really distinct can be inseparable." Beyond what Deleuze states, it is possible to use the idea that in a relationship, the elements, from which a structure emerges, can be thought of as distinct and inseparable. This approach is opposite to what happens in combinatorial interaction. Inseparability refers to the fact that, although the elements of a system are distinct, they are defined, have meaning and function only within a relationship. For this reason, they should be considered "inseparable." This characterization allows us to understand the emergence of complex properties and phenomena (Marinucci, 2023).

This aspect is very important because the possibilities of a structure, not predeterminable a priori, also assume a certain configuration, depending on the way in which a relationship is actually configured and the scientific question at stake (e.g., it is different to ask questions about gene expression or functional question regarding proteins activities; or to ask a question about the chemical effect of a food on a specific molecular receptor or a functional/physiological effect in the liver of a baby or of an adult). The configurations and properties that a phenomenon can show certainly refer to the difference that emerges in a specific relationship regarding an organismic determination of the object. From this point of view, "explaining" a phenomenon does not mean achieving a complete and objective vision.

On the contrary, the more perspectives there are of an object, the more the "objectivity" of knowledge increases.

Relations and inseparability constitute different levels and interfaces in which to consider a property or a phenomenon. The difficulties in identifying a precise linear causal regime configure causality as complex. In other words, if causes exist, these act in a relational way, co-constituting and co-implicating each other.

Life's knowledge is always contextual. There are never the necessary and sufficient conditions for someone to get sick. In biology, it is not always sufficient for a cause to exist for it to be active. Everyone has pathogens (viruses and bacteria) in their organism, but one is not always sick: often in biology, causes have to be activated to manifest themselves. Diseases can be considered as emergent phenomena, linked to a specific type of organic relationship that makes the manifestation of a disease possible and real (Ilardo & Bertolaso, 2024).

The choice of the level of description allows us to manage this uncertainty locally. It is therefore possible to manage a problem related to a disease or a complex social issue. The more levels and interfaces of a phenomenon are discovered, the more it is known and can be managed, considering that these are complex objects. It is precisely from the characterization of an epistemology of complexity that the need for an epistemology of uncertainty emerges. Although it cannot define something in a complete and objective way, it allows the management of complex objects, giving the tools of scientific investigation their own epistemological status. After all, complexity arises precisely on the limits of determinism, reductionism.

Object of Knowledge and Real Object

In a Relational Perspective, the Object of Knowledge and Real Object Never Coincide, Precisely because Multiple Perspectives on the Real Object Are Possible (Mitchell, 2009; Agazzi, 2021). The Main Element Is However another. Within this Perspective, both Formal and Content Constraints Do Not Apply. First of all, the Non-coincidence between Object of Knowledge and Real Object Makes it Possible to Build Multiple Ontologies Linked to the Level of Knowledge that Illuminate Aspects of the Real Object. As Regards the Formal Constraint, Knowledge Can Be Structured in a Plural Way, without Absolute Fundamental Explanatory Levels. They Are Linked to Criteria of Relevance. In this Way, when there Is a Complex Causality, Scientific and Methodological Tools Will Constitute Adequate Objects of Knowledge with their Own Epistemological Status, without Having to Presuppose a Fundamental Level of Explanatory Certainty. Therefore, the Object of Knowledge Represents (it Is Not) the Real Object for a Specific Purpose, for a Specific Knowledge. In Other Words, it Constitutes an Interpretation of it, Linked to a Point of View. It Is Important to Emphasize that this Characterization of the Object of Knowledge and the Real Object Does Not Fall into Relativism. In Fact, if the Problem to Be Solved Is a Disease, the Constitution of the Object of Knowledge Refers to that Specific Level, through Criteria of Relevance. It Is Different to Deal with a Cold than with Cancer

The object of knowledge is not the real object. It allows us to interpret the real object, constituting specific interfaces to describe properties and phenomena, so that they can be managed, since they cannot be controlled.

Especially in biology and social sciences, another element that determines the difference between a real object and an object of knowledge is that the real object changes over time. This type of object has a history in which it constantly changes, while maintaining a constitutive relational structure. For example, organisms change over time. The change is obviously ontophylogenetically constrained, but the specific forms it can take are not determinable, because they are emergent. Two identical twins have different fingerprints and a different biographical and ontogenetic history. It seems clear that in this case the formal and content constraints are not applicable, but a relational approach is necessary, focusing on the constitution of the object of knowledge, on the specific case. That is, the contingent and contextual feature constitutes the most interesting object of inquiry. Existing mathematical tools are unable to describe the dynamics of the changing object. They are able to describe the object that moves, maintaining its contingent empirical features.

Uncertainty, Risk and Perception of Science

The Epistemology of Certainty and the Epistemology of Uncertainty Address Two Different Situations in which it Is Necessary to Make Decisions. As Seen, in the Case of Certainty, Science Is Able to Provide Certain Answers. In this Case, there Are no Problems. In the Case of the Epistemology of Uncertainty, there Is an Epistemological Basis for Being Able to Base Decisions when there Are no Certainties, I.E., Considering the Conditions under which the Different Possibilities of a Living System Can Reveal itself. Not Being Able to Control a Phenomenon Does Not Mean that it Is Not Possible to Act. It Is Possible to Give an Epistemological Status to the Tools that Allow us to Manage Uncertainty. This Is Essential in Politics and Law because in these Areas it Is Always Necessary to Make Decisions

As we will see with regard to the precautionary principle, in the legal field uncertainty is not yet considered as something from which it is possible to decide. In fact, the application of precaution occurs when there is no certainty, but, after a period of time, it is not maintained if there is no certain evidence. When uncertainty becomes certainty, then it is really necessary to revoke the precautionary principle. If uncertainty remains, it is necessary to manage it and the resulting risks.[14]

This situation is linked to complex causality, so it is not possible to predict what configuration a phenomenon will have. However, it is

---

[14] From a philosophical point of view, the most important elements are 1. There are situations of uncertainty, 2. there are scientific tools to manage uncertainty, 3 these tools do not have their own epistemological status. The consequence of 3. is that definitive decisions cannot be made starting from the tools to manage uncertainty (2.).

possible to make decisions starting from the identification of the level at which a phenomenon can be studied, i.e., from the construction of an object of knowledge and focusing on its specific constitutive relationships. Probability and the tools to deal with uncertainty and risk have to have their own epistemological status. In the previous pages, some epistemological tools have been exposed such as the distinction between real object and object of knowledge, complex causality, the concept of relationship, etc. Now it is necessary to mention some scientific analysis tools whose results can be given an epistemological status.

Risk is defined as an undesirable event or condition, characterized by uncertainty and the possibility of variable outcomes in the future (Rosa 1998). This concept is closely linked to causality, which influences the perception of risk and the decisions to be made. According to ISO 31000 (2018), risk is "the effect of uncertainty on objectives." It can include both positive and negative deviations from an expected result. Risk management is therefore essential to reduce the impact of adverse events, through the analysis of possible causes and mitigation strategies (Aven & Zio, 2014; Aven, 2016; SRA, 2015).

Since uncertainty is an inevitable part of risk management, it is necessary to develop effective strategies to deal with it. A static and rigid approach to risk management is not enough. It is necessary to adopt dynamic and adaptive methodologies that can respond to constantly evolving scenarios. One of the most effective ways to reduce uncertainty is to use predictive models and simulations. These tools allow us to test different scenarios and evaluate the effect of various risk factors. The underlying problem is that risk is linked to causality, which is complex: it is not always possible to establish a direct and proportional link between cause and effect.[15]

After identifying risks, it is necessary to develop strategies to reduce their effects. Risk management is based on a preventive approach, which involves reducing the probability of an adverse event occurring and preparing to respond effectively in the event of an emergency (Iqbal,

[15] From this point of view, the distance mentioned between Laplace and Poincaré is exemplary. In the history of scientific thought, it recurs in other forms, but substantially does not change.

2019). In these cases, it is essential to identify the appropriate levels and interfaces.

The first step of risk analysis consists in identifying potential hazards and assessing their impact. This step is essential to understand the probability of a harmful event occurring and to estimate its consequences. Risk identification can be done through different methods, for example historical analysis, predictive models and experiential assessments (Anjum & Rocca, 2019). However, uncertainty plays a key role in this step, since it is not always possible to obtain complete and reliable data.

Nonetheless, the analyses proper to an epistemology of uncertainty lead to focusing attention on elements that are relevant in a given context. In this way, it is possible to reduce the risk and better construct the object of knowledge, allowing for better management of complexity.

In order to go beyond the limits of determinism and reductionism, new models have been developed that combine different epistemological perspectives. Among these, the Bayesian approach represents an important methodological innovation, allowing updating beliefs on the basis of new evidence and to manage uncertainty in a more flexible way. According to Pearl (2009) and Hitchcock (2016), Bayesian models allow representing causal interactions through probabilistic networks, which take into account complex interactions between variables and allow adapting inferences in response to new data. This approach has been applied in numerous sectors, from medicine to environmental risk management, to improve decision-making strategies under uncertainty. Another emerging approach is the concept of systemic resilience, which emphasizes the ability of a system to adapt to unexpected changes rather than trying to predict and control every possible event. In this case, the focus shifts from deterministic prediction to managing complexity through flexible and adaptive strategies.

These examples are extremely interesting because they represent concrete tools for managing complexity. Obviously, there are many others. They are different depending on the context in which they are applied: biology, medicine, law, sociology, etc. What was necessary was to provide an epistemological basis able to associate these and other tools with their own epistemological status. In fact, their results do not always have to be conceived starting from a certainty. As mentioned, complexity has to be addressed in itself, because the resulting indeterminacy is not always reducible or eliminable. For this reason, it was necessary to clearly show the part of reality to which complex phenomena and their characteristics of uncertainty (often intrinsic) refer.

In this sense, it is not just a matter of placing several methods side by side, presupposing a homogeneous, unique, open and undifferentiated conceptual space from which to choose. It is a matter of reflecting on the fact that it is this same conceptual space that is the object of construction and that it is always subject to modifications, when a definition is constructed. The aim is precisely to maintain a plurality of co-present perspectives and to avoid surreptitiously binding the possibility to any closed and self-referential rationality.

Complex causality, risk, uncertainty, probability, etc. can now be used in the legal and political spheres (and not only) to make decisions, without the need for a scientific certainty. Where there is the latter, then it is possible to decide within an epistemology of certainty. Where this is not possible, it is necessary to use the epistemology of uncertainty.

According to Giampietro and Saltelli (Benessia et al., 2016), uncertainty is intrinsic to science and politics. It is often hidden to create an illusion of certainty in decision-making processes. They criticize scientific reductionism that leads to simplifying complex problems through quantitative models that ignore the plurality of relevant factors (Rayner, 2012; p. 41). An example is the fallacy of economic models, which have erroneously predicted the stability of markets based on simplified and linearized hypotheses (Saltelli et al., 2013). This type of error is amplified by the lack of mathematical analysis on the stability of economic systems. This leads to a wrong perception of the safety of decisions based on mathematical models.

In the application of the precautionary principle, the same assumption applies, based on an epistemology of certainty. In other words, it is possible to decide only on certainties (Manson, 2013). In the following pages, the precautionary principle in the food sector will be discussed, but what will be said also applies to other uses of this principle, for example in the field of environmental sustainability.[16]

4 The Precautionary Principle

There are different formulations of the precautionary principle. These can be divided into two legal categories: soft law and hard law. In the first case, these are legal instruments that, despite being normative, do not have direct binding force. In fact, they have a guiding function also and not only in the interpretation of hard law norms. The latter are characterized by the fact that they are binding norms, such as civil rights. In Europe the precautionary principle is hard law, while in the rest of the world it is soft law.

The European precautionary principle states:

Precautionary principle

1. In specific circumstances where, following an assessment of available information, the possibility of harmful effects on health is identified but scientific uncertainty persists, provisional risk management measures necessary to ensure the high level of health protection chosen in the Community may be adopted, pending further scientific information for a more comprehensive risk assessment.
2. Measures adopted on the basis of paragraph 1 shall be proportionate and no more restrictive of trade than is required to achieve the high level of health protection chosen in the Community, regard being had to technical and economic feasibility and other factors regarded as legitimate in the matter under consideration. The measures shall be reviewed within a reasonable period of time, depending on the nature

[16] In general, the precautionary principle is discussed mainly in the environmental field (Gardiner, 2006; Weiss, 2003). However, there are no relevant differences in the debate regarding its use in food.

of the risk to life or health identified and the type of scientific information needed to clarify the scientific uncertainty and to conduct a more comprehensive risk assessment.[17]

Two examples of formulations of the precautionary principle concerning the environment, often cited (Gardiner, 2006; Weiss, 2003), in the soft law regime are the following. The Rio de Janeiro Declaration (1992) states:

> In order to protect the environment, the precautionary principle shall be widely applied by States according to their capabilities. Where there are threats of serious or irreversible damage, lack of full scientific certainty shall not be used as a reason for postponing cost-effective measures to prevent environmental degradation (United Nations, 1992, p. 10) (Resnik, 2003).

The Wingspread Declaration (1998) states:

> When an activity raises threats of harm to human health or the environment, precautionary measures should be taken even if some cause and effect relationships are not fully established scientifically. [...]. In this context the proponent of an activity, rather than the public bears the burden of proof.

The difference between the two examples is that the second requires the adoption of precautionary rules. The European Commission (1987) specifies that each state has "the right to establish the level it deems appropriate" (Weiss, 2003), thus expressing the idea that it is necessary to consider the particularity of situations in the application of the precautionary principle.

Outside Europe, the precautionary principle does not have the same strength as in Europe, but there are important similarities. In general,

---

[17] Regulation (EC) No 178/2002 of the European Parliament and of the Council of 28 January 2002 laying down the general principles and requirements of food law, establishing the European Food Safety Authority and laying down procedures in matters of food safety. https://eur-lex.europa.eu/eli/reg/2002/178/oj/eng

the precautionary principle is applied to foods to block them in case of health risks.

More precisely, if food products, before being marketed, are considered dangerous a priori by the legislator, the "principle of preventive authorization" is applied (Bruno, 2017). In this case, it is the producer who has to scientifically demonstrate that his products do not present health risks. This case does not create major legal problems, because legislation exists and the product is not yet marketed. If it is already on the market and if the possibility of health risks arises, the precautionary principle can be applied.[18] In this case, the burden of proof of the risk passes to the institutions.

The crucial problem is that if after a certain period of time the harmfulness or non-harmfulness of the food is not demonstrated, it is put back on the market (Bruno, 2017, Bruno, 2000). Analyzing the reasoning scheme of the application and maintenance of the precautionary principle, a contradiction appears. It can be resolved by applying the proposed distinction between epistemology of certainty and epistemology of uncertainty.

1. The principle applies when a food on the market presents or may present health problems
2. There is uncertainty at the basis of its application.
3. In order to maintain the food block, the certainty of its harmfulness is necessary.

The short circuit arises because it is not always possible to move from uncertainty to certainty. Furthermore, if the principle is applied when there is no certainty, it is not always possible to require certainty to continue and maintain it. Wherever certainty is reached, the situation is resolved. The contradiction arises because science is perceived as always being able to provide certainties. This derives from the fact that definitive decisions are taken only within an epistemology of certainty. The precautionary principle is an excellent example to show the need to be

[18] It should be emphasized that, since the product is already on the market, it is normally taken action when some health problem arises.

able to decide starting from an epistemology of uncertainty. In fact, if the harmfulness of a food is not demonstrated, there is no certainty that it is not harmful to health.

Starting from what was said in the first part of this paper, a new way of thinking is needed. It has to allow decisions to be made based on different criteria, when necessary. These criteria are dependent on the context and on the possibility of making definitive[19] decisions based on the management of uncertainty. For example, in the formulations of the precautionary principle it is clear that decisions, based on uncertainty, can only be provisional (Bruno, 2017).

The Philosophical Debate

With Respect to the Philosophical Debate on the Precautionary Principle, no Author Proposes an Epistemology of Uncertainty to Conceive this Issue Differently. In the Last Section of this Paper, it Will Be Seen that the Moral Concept of Precaution Must Have a Different Epistemological Basis for its Complete Application and for its Maintenance. In General, there Is Discussion about the Formulations of the Precautionary Principle, Trying to Improve them. In some Cases, Solutions Are Proposed without Providing an Epistemological Basis. This Is What Legitimizes the Use of the Tools (as Probability, Risk Management) that Manage Uncertainty and that Give it an Epistemological Status (Gardiner, 2006). This Step Is Crucial because Recognizing an Epistemological Status Is the Basis for Making Even Definitive Decisions on Precautionary Measures

In the literature on the subject (for example: Bodansky, 1991; Gardiner, 2006; Lemons, et al. 1997; Manson, 2013; Resnik, 2003; Sandin et al., 2013; Steglich-Petersen, 2015; Tallacchini, 2005; Weiss, 2003), there is a certain insistence on complete and formally perfect

---

[19] The use of the adjective "definitive" is due to the fact that the precautionary principle applies only provisionally. In this paper, it will be shown that it is possible to apply it for "definitive" decisions only if the management of uncertainty has its own epistemological status (when science does not provide certainty).

definitions[20] of the precautionary principle. This often leads to forgetting that it is not always necessary to go uncritically in the direction of a complete definition (Wittgenstein, 1999b). As seen, in cases where uncertainty prevails, the definition (what) comes after the description (how) of a phenomenon. Nonetheless, if an adequate definition of the precautionary principle remains necessary, it is necessary to understand what kind of formulation such principle requires. Again, preliminary philosophical work is necessary. It is not trivial to underline that the precautionary principle is, in fact, a "principle." A principle is not something that applies directly to concrete cases,[21] but is that with respect to which a theory, a legal corpus, etc. is built. Borrowing a Kantian expression, it is what with respect to which thought is oriented (Kant, 1996). It has a regulative function on the basis of which laws can be written that will be applied to concrete cases. In this sense, the fact that the European definition is hard law, obliges the legislator and the jurist to create the prerequisites and structures for a de facto application of the precaution. Considering the different fields in which this principle can be applied, what has been said is even more important. In fact, they require the creation of a system that integrates biology, medicine and law.

It is necessary to reiterate these aspects because the formulations of the precautionary principle are accused of not containing obligations or of containing too few and of being written in a negative form.[22]

In reality, a single and general formulation would be really needed: a principle has the function of orienting legislation and its applications to real cases. What does "orient" mean in this case? A couple of examples. If only the principle of economic gain existed, environmental and human health issues would be subordinated only to a cost analysis. Thus,

---

20 "Definition" comes from "finis" which means border.

21 Some authors fall into an overlapping of conceptual levels (Bodansky, 2004).

22 This type of formulation is normal, but in the texts mentioned the discussion between positive and negative formulation is present. In general, all principles are stated negatively, because there are many ways to act coherently with them. Only in the case in which the object of the principle is concrete, a positive formulation can be given, but in this case the indeterminacy of the principle consists in 'how' to reach the objective. Regardless of the definitions that may be more or less strong, it is important to remember that outside Europe the precautionary principle falls within soft law.

it would also be possible to act to safeguard nature, but in the background the principle of economic gain would always remain, prevailing, precisely because the latter orients choices. Furthermore, trying to think of a society based on a principle of violence or racism, the orientation of action would be differently characterized; just look at the history of the twentieth century. The strongest opponents of the precautionary principle claim that in reality one wants to block scientific progress (Gardiner, 2006).

The very fact that a principle guides implies the need to analyze concrete cases to make a decision. The precautionary principle expresses caution, then it is the laws and concrete cases that may or may not contain prohibitions.

It is important to underline—although beyond the possibility of a proper discussion in this paper—that the possible fundamental clash of the application of the precautionary principle is quite often profit vs. health. In this regard, the precautionary principle seeks a mediation and a conciliation between these two elements, orienting toward health.

Some Morals

The function of a principle is to orient the choices and decisions that are made in practice. Therefore, it has certainly to be general (Bodansky, 2004; Manson, 2013), but it has to have the strength to orient the jurist and the politician. A clear example of what is meant is represented by the difference between constitutional laws and ordinary laws. The former set out the general principles to which other laws must conform.

In the specific case of the precautionary principle, it orients toward the protection of health. Prioritizing health can mean many things, for this reason the precautionary principle has to have a general definition that will be filled in from time to time.

This aspect is very important because “precaution” is first and foremost a moral concept, which has to be applied within the law. From this point of view, precaution has to be considered as a form of rationality[23] rather than as something that regulates. The norm is legal and is set in the contingency of the specific areas in which the precautionary principle is applied. "Form of rationality" means that precaution and health represent the horizon of meaning within which the debates and analyses of concrete cases on the application of the principle should move. In this sense, the precautionary principle, in the cases in which it is applied, orients action toward health. A principle can be thought of as a form of operational rationality, as a moral concept. The fact that it is an operational rationality means that it is not merely speculative. It has to lead to behaviors that conform to the form of rationality to which they refer. Secondly, from a legal point of view, this has to lead to the production of specific laws that give concreteness and consistency to the precautionary principle. In order to move from the moral sphere to the legal sphere, it is necessary to find one or more connections between these two spheres.

The link between precaution and the legal sphere is certainly given by the fact that there are legal formulations that qualify it as a principle, but it also resides in another element: health. Now, if precaution is a "principle" (soft or hard law), health is a right,[24] at least in Western constitutions. In a very general way, if health is a right (and is a priority in the Italian legal system), then laws and political decisions have to favor the right to health. In the specific case of nutrition and the situation in which the precautionary principle is applied, the question of health immediately becomes fundamental. In the application and maintenance of precautionary measures, it is a question of mediating between health and economic gain. If the precautionary principle is a form of expression of the right to health, determining the horizon of operational rationality within which the politician and the jurist have to move, then it can assume even more strength in the formulation of laws.

The link between the precautionary principle and the right to health allows it to be strengthened, but does not solve the problem of its

[23] This expression underlines and translates operationally a practical reasoning on the model of Aristotle (Aristotle 2003, § VI, 2), see (Natali 1984; Natali 1989). Obviously, here we have taken only inspiration from Aristotle's text, without claiming to discuss it in detail.

[24] It is not trivial to remember that Article 25 of the Universal Declaration of Human Rights recognizes health as a right.

maintenance. It is useful to remember that if the harmfulness or non-harmfulness of the food is not demonstrated, after a period of time, it is put back on the market. This is based on a logic of certainty, whereby decisions are made only on the basis of certainties. This aspect implies that only certainty has its own epistemological status. In other words, only certainty legitimizes the taking of legal and/or political decisions.

Alongside the world of certainties, there is a world of uncertainties that can also be unsolvable. It is necessary to know how to manage this world and be able to decide even in these cases. Therefore, the crucial point is epistemological because sophisticated tools already exist to manage uncertainty. It is a question of giving these tools their own epistemological status, beyond the epistemology of certainty. If an epistemological status is granted to the epistemology of uncertainty, then it is possible to legitimize even definitive decisions on food starting from criteria that are not scientific certainty. Obviously, this occurs in cases where there is no scientific certainty. Prudence becomes in these cases the ethical counterpart of the constitutive uncertainty and relational ontology that characterizes the living systems and dynamics.

The tools for managing uncertainty have already been mentioned. These are already used within science. However, for their different application and valorization, they should be conceived within an epistemology of uncertainty. In this way, it will be possible to make definitive decisions. Thus, the perception of science in the legal and political fields can change. The separation between the object of knowledge and the real object and the concept of relationship allow the passage to an epistemology of uncertainty and from control to management, without necessarily having to presuppose a fundamental certainty.

References

Agazzi, E. (2021). *La conoscenza dell'invisibile*. MIMESIS Edizioni.

Anjum, R.L., Rocca, E. (2019), From ideal to real risk: philosophy of causation meets risk analysis, *In Risk Analysis, 39*, pp. 729–740.

Aristotle. (2003). *Etica Nicomachea*. Bompiani.

Arora, M., Giuliani, A., & Curtin, P. (2020). Biodynamic interfaces are essential for human–environment interactions. *Bio Essays, 42*(11), e2000017.

Aven, T. (2016), Risk assessment and risk management: Review of recent advances on their foundation, *In European Journal of Operational Research, 253* (1), pp. 1–13.

Aven, T. & Zio, E. (2014), Foundational issues in risk assessment and risk management, *In Risk Analysis, 34*(7), pp. 1164–1172.

Bailly, F. & Longo, G. (2006). Mathématiques et sciences de la nature. Paris: Hermann. Eng. Transl. (2011) *Mathematics and the natural sciences; The Physical Singularity of Life*. Imperial College Press.

Barrow-Green, J. (1997). Poincaré and the three body problem. *American Mathematical Society, 11.*

Benessia, A., Funtowicz, S., Giampietro, M., Pereira, Â. G., Ravetz, J. R., Saltelli, A., & Van der Sluijs, J. P. (2016). *The Rightful Place of Science. Science on the Verge*. Tempe, AZ Consortium for Science, Policy & Outcomes. https://books.google.it/books?id=bjGVjwEACAAJ

Bertolaso, M. (2013a). La indeterminación biológica y las perspectivas sistémicas de la biología contemporánea. *Anuario filosófico, 46*(2), 365–386.

Bertolaso, M. (2013b). *How science works: Choosing levels of explanation in biological sciences*. Aracne.

Bertolaso, M. (2016). *Philosophy of cancer. A dynamic and relational view*. Springer.

Bertolaso, M., & Kovacic, Z. (2024). *Narrative per una società consapevole*. Rubbettino.

Bertolaso, M., & Marinucci, A. (2024). *Le questioni aperte della vita*. Rubbettino.

Bocchi, G., & Ceruti, M. (Eds.). (2007). *La sfida della complessità*. Bruno Mondadori.

Bodansky, D. (1991). Law: Scientific uncertainty and the precautionary principle. *Environment: Science and Policy for Sustainable Development, 33*(7), 4–44. https://doi.org/10.1080/00139157.1991.9929978

Bodansky, D. (2004). Deconstructing the precautionary principle. In D. D. Caron & H. N. Scheiber (Eds.), *Bringing new law to ocean waters* (pp. 381–391). Brill.

Bruno, F. (2000). Il principio di precauzione tra diritto dell'Unione Europea e WTO. *Diritto E Giurisprudenza Agraria E Dellambiente, 569*.

Bruno, F. (2017). *Il diritto alimentare nel contesto globale: USA e UE a confronto*. Wolters Kluwer.

Cini, M. (1999). *Un paradiso perduto*. Feltrinelli.

Darwin, C. (1859) The origin of species.

Deleuze, G. (2004). *La piega. Leibniz e il barocco.* Einaudi.

Descartes, R. (2000). *Regole per la guida dell'intelligenza.* Bompiani.

Dupré, J., & Nicholson, J. (2018). A manifesto for a processual philosophy of biology. In J. Dupré & J. Nicholson (Eds.), *Everything flows: Towards a processual philosophy of biology.* Oxford University Press.

Euler, L. (1960a). Recherches sur la question des inégalités du mouvement de Saturn et de Jupiter. In *Leonhardi Euleri Opera omnia.* 2, 25. Lipsia.

Euler, L. (1960b). Recherches sur le mouvement des corps célestes en général. In *Leonhardi Euleri Opera omnia* (Vol. 2, p. 25). Lipsia.

Gardiner, S. M. (2006). A Core precautionary principle. *The Journal of Political Philosophy, 14*(1), 33–60. https://doi.org/10.1111/j.1467-9760.2006.00237

Hitchcock, C. (2016). Probabilistic causation. In A. Hájek & C. Hitchcock (Eds.), *The Oxford handbook of probability and philosophy* (pp. 815–832). Oxford University Press.

Ilardo, M. L., & Bertolaso, M. (2024). Exploring the interplay of causality notions & risk concepts: Epistemological implications. *Teoria. Rivista di filosofia, 44*(1).

Iqbal, M. (2019), Known Risks and Unknown Risk, MI, http://siriqbal.net/known-risk-and-unknown-risks/.

Israel, G. (1991). Il determinismo e la teoria delle equazioni differenziali ordinarie. *Physis, 28*, 305–358.

Kant, I. (1996). *Che cosa significa orientarsi nel pensiero.* Adelphi.

Laplace, P. S. (1967). Saggio sulla probabilità delle cause in base agli avvenimenti. In *Opere.* UTET.

Lemons, J., Shrader-Frechette, K., & Cranor, C. (1997). The precautionary principle: Scientific uncertainty and type I and type II errors. *Foundations of Science, 2*(2), 207–236.

Manson, N. A. (2013). Formulating the precautionary principle. In A. Bird & J. Ladyman (Eds.), *Arguing about science* (pp. 607–616). Routledge.

Marinucci, A. (2011). *Tra ordine e caos. Metodi e linguaggi tra fisica, matematica e filosofia.* Aracne.

Marinucci, A. (2023). *Theoretical principles of relational biology.* Springer.

Mitchell, S. D. (2009). *Unsimple truths: Science, complexity and policy.* University of Chicago Press.

Morin, E. (2007). Le vie della complessità. In *La sfida della complessità. A cura di Bocchi Gianluca e Mauro Ceruti.* Bruno Mondadori.

Natali, C. (1984). Virtù o scienza? Aspetti della phronesis nei Topici e nelle Etiche di Aristotele. *Phronesis, 1*(29), 50–72.

Natali, C. (1989). *La saggezza di Aristotele*. Bibliopolis.
Paty, M. (1988). D'Alembert et les probabilités. In R. Rashed (Ed.), *Sciences à l'époque de la Révolution française. Recherches historiques*. Blanchard. 203–265.
Pearl, J. (2009). *Causality: Models, reasoning, and inference* (2nd ed.). Cambridge University Press.
Poincaré, H. (2006). Il problema dei tre corpi. In A. Bartocci (Ed.), *Geometria e caos*. Bollati Boringhieri.
Rayner, S. (2012). Uncomfortable knowledge: The social construction of ignorance in science and environmental policy discourses. *Economy and Society, 41*(1), 107–125.
Regulation (EC) No 178/2002 of the European Parliament and of the Council of 28 January. 2002. Laying down the general principles and requirements of food law, establishing the European Food Safety Authority and laying down procedures in matters of food safety. https://eur-lex.europa.eu/eli/reg/2002/178/oj/eng
Resnik, D. B. (2003). Is the precautionary principle unscientific? *Studies in History and Philosophy of Science Part C: Studies in History and Philosophy of Biological and Biomedical Sciences, 34*(2), 329–344.
Saltelli, A., Guimarães Pereira, A., van der Sluijs, J. P. & Funtowicz, S., 2013. What do I make of your Latinorum? Sensitivity auditing of mathematical modelling, *International Journal of Foresight and Innovation Policy, 9*(2–4): 213–234.
Sandin, P., et al. (2013). Five charges against the precautionary principle. In A. Bird & J. Ladyman (Eds.), *Arguing about science* (pp. 617–628). Routledge.
SRA. (2015), *Risk Analysis Foundations, Society for Risk Analysis*. https://li338–15.members.linode.com/news/discussion-paper-foundations-risk-analysis-developed-sra; https://www.sra.org/wp-content/uploads/FRASG/FoundationsMay7-2015-sent-x.pdf.
Steglich-Petersen, A. (2015). The epistemology of the precautionary principle: Two puzzles resolved. *Erkenntnis, 80*, 1013–1021. https://doi.org/10.1007/s10670-014-9694-x
Stengers, I. (2007). Perché non può esserci un paradigma della complessità. In G. Bocchi & M. Ceruti (Eds.), *La sfida della complessità*. Bruno Mondadori.
Tabor, M. (1989). *Chaos and Integrability in nonlinear dynamics*. John Wiley & Sons.
Tallacchini, M. (2005). Before and beyond the precautionary principle: Epistemology of uncertainty in science and law. *Toxicology and Applied Pharmacology, 207*(2), 645–651. https://doi.org/10.1016/j.taap.2004.12.029

Weaver W. (1948). Science and complexity Classical Papers. *Science and complexity* E:CO Vol. 6 No. 3 2004, 65–74.

Weiss, C. (2003). Scientific uncertainty and science-based precaution. *International Environmental Agreements: Politics, Law and Economics, 137–166*. https://doi.org/10.1023/A:1024847807590

Wells, J. (2011). *The myth of junk DNA* (Vol. 85). Discovery Institute Press.

Wimsatt, W. C. (2007). *Re-engineering philosophy for limited beings: Piecewise approximations to reality*. Harvard University Press.

Wittgenstein, L. (1999a). *Libro blu e libro marrone*. Einaudi.

Wittgenstein, L. (1999b). *Ricerche filosofiche*. Einaudi.

The Great Acceleration and the Biopolitics of Nutrition

Roger Strand

1 Introduction

This book chapter was born out of a request for a reflection on science, nutrition advice and how people eat, in particular in modern societies in the twenty-first century, and more specifically on the role of scientific uncertainty. Can Science tell us what we should eat? And if not, why not?

My original reply to this request might be seen as slightly off topic. Rather than giving another exposition of scientific uncertainty, I was led to reflect on biopolitics, on sustainability challenges, and what in the world of environmental and sustainability governance has been called "the Great Acceleration". It led me to write a prospect, a kind of extended

R. Strand (✉)
Centre for the Study of the Sciences and the Humanities, University of Bergen, Bergen, Norway
e-mail: roger.strand@uib.no

F. Bruno et al. (eds.), *Healthcare and Food*,
https://doi.org/10.1007/978-981-95-5899-5_2

abstract as the point of departure. It is a sweeping gesture of contemporary history. I will share it so that readers can get a quick idea of where this chapter is going. Here it comes:

The Industrial Revolution laid the foundation for two dramatic changes in the human condition. It set off sociotechnical trajectories of exponential growth in human production and consumption in what has been called the Great Acceleration. On the one hand, this offered unprecedented technological capabilities at the individual and collective level. On the other, it led to unprecedented environmental problems and risks to the extent that sustainability science feared irreversible collapse of ecological and socio-ecological systems. Simultaneously, as part of these sociotechnical trajectories, a new form of politics arose by which it became a legitimate concern of the modern state to govern the size of its human population and the health state of its individual subjects. In this development of biopolitics and biopower, medicine, nutrition science and food science came to play important roles. With the very best intentions, these sciences have developed within a logic of control-and-command and with hopes of governing human populations towards long, healthy, productive and well-nourished lives.

Moving into the second quarter of the twenty-first century, the anomalies and fractures in the modern world are increasingly visible. The Great Acceleration cannot continue much longer. The Earth is becoming full of us, our waste and our livestock as we pollute and deplete natural resources. Modern biopolitical orders are cracking up into violent, non-or post-humanitarian disorder, now also in the Global North. Within protected elites, utopian imaginaries of perfect health and nutrition are still cultivated together with equally utopian hopes in sciences of certainty and control. In the larger picture, however, these elites are both becoming irrelevant and paradoxically also strong drivers of the escalating conflicts and fractures.

It is time to think. What sciences will be sorely needed in the post-growth era, after the Great Acceleration? Which conceptualisations of food and the good life will humans need to flourish after the downfall of biopolitics of nutrition and health?

How does one create a book chapter from this possibly pompous statement?—pompous in the sense of pretending to be able to know what is the general state of the world, and then again only *possibly* pompous if the author is able to deliver it with reflexivity, with an awareness that it is a partial story, an experiment in developing an argument from a set of premises, an *assay* in the true sense.

Indeed, how to write? This is a methodological question which in the period of writing of this book underwent a radical change. In 2022, the company OpenAI released its chatbot "ChatGPT" for (partially) free use on the internet. In the year of writing this book, 2025, the so-called AI boom had made ChatGPT, Microsoft Copilot and a number of other chatbot-based AI services ubiquitous tools for academics and lay citizens alike, not the least in the Global North. As a Norwegian university professor, I witnessed how work life changed in 2024 and 2025. Students had to be warned or advised or guided to write themselves and not simply get the bots to write for them (and of course they often used the bots anyway). As if we full-time professional academics did not use these tools ourselves.

Hence, in 2025, one way to answer the question of how to write the current book chapter was simply to ask the chatbot. So, I did. I ran the extended abstract just presented, by Microsoft Copilot, which immediately proposed a book chapter with 8 parts. The three first were:

1. Introduction, with an overview of the Great Acceleration, stating the purpose and scope of the chapter and defining key questions.
2. Historical Foundations, introducing the Industrial Revolution and the concept of sociotechnical trajectories, and explaining how there has been exponential growth in production and consumption.
3. Biopolitics and the Modern State, introducing Foucault's concept of biopolitics and biopower, before discussing the role(s) of medicine, nutrition science, and food science, and how there is a dominant control-and-command logic in public health and nutrition.

Following this, Microsoft Copilot wanted me to describe ongoing environmental degradation and ecological limits; socio-political instability; and then the illusion of control in elite utopias. Next, present characteristics of a post-Great Acceleration world, challenges and opportunities for governance and science, and the possible decline of biopolitical paradigms. And then finally, I ought to develop the argument of "rethinking food and nutrition", moving from a focus on nutrition science to food studies that study food cultures, traditions, and the good life, and then more largely reimagining health, well-being, and sustainability. The chatbot ended with generously asking if I would like help "drafting any specific section of the chapter or finding sources to support your arguments".

In 2025, my colleagues and I used the chatbot in this way—as a toy residing somewhere in the uncanny valley, as a way to explore its capacities, get some ideas and perhaps laugh and make the joke that now we can all retire. And indeed, after contemplating the outline that the chatbot presented and not the least its offer to draft the entire text, I concluded that I should retire from this kind of scholarship, this way of being a good boy, as it were, to step-by-step delineate and expound on the topic I had set forth. We do not need humans for this kind of text anymore. Future readers of this book, who are likely to read it in some digital format, can just copy the chapter title or the passage in italics—the "point of departure"—themselves and paste it into a prompt of their favourite AI chatbot, and they will certainly get a smoother, more balanced and better informed text than anything this author can write.

So, we human authors are now set free. We no longer have to be good boys or girls. We can do something more important. Following Deleuze and Guattarí (and of course many others), we can rather develop new thoughts and concepts to open up new plans for action (Deleuze & Guattari, 1994). We can devote ourselves to *think*, this important activity that humans can engage in and that sets us apart from the chatbots. Chatbots based on large language models do not think, they produce outputs predicted by their language model to be appropriate to the corresponding inputs. In the case of popular, widespread chatbots, such as Microsoft Copilot, I expect that the appropriateness of their outputs somehow is also validated by their users, in the sense that they match their general expectations. Otherwise, one might expect public outcries, complaints or decreasing use. Indeed, by 2025, this had become an issue—when users found a particular update of a chatbot too flattering or too impersonal or too unreliable.

Specifically, I had personally experienced how ChatGPT and Microsoft Copilot outputs seemed to share three features:

1. They were (mostly) *on topic*. They stayed within the realm of concept and phenomena that were introduced to them by the input.
2. They were *polite*. Unless specifically prompted to, they refrained from making claims that could be perceived as highly critical, provoking or uncomfortable to whoever uttered the original input or suggested the initial topic.
3. They were *predictable*. They stayed within some dominant or distinct *discourse* indicated to them by the prompt (within the safe limits of the ethical and political boundaries and constraints programmed into their algorithms). If prompted with a (moderately) strong ideological statement, they would respond more to this kind of talk. If the author of a query showed a strong belief in science, they would return and confirm it. If she or he instead displayed a clear critical stand, the bot would reproduce arguments and tropes from a more critical discourse. Not being an LLM expert, I assume that this is a consequence of their language models being large: They are trained on so much text that their output is excellent at being mainstream within the particular part of the text universe they find themselves in at any given moment.

My methodological conclusion was accordingly clear: We humans may now do the opposite of staying on topic and being polite and predictable. The kind of texts that human scholars now are free to write, and perhaps even should prioritise to write, may explore exactly the liberties that are denied to the chatbots. We may allow ourselves to jump between, combine and fertilise discourses and challenge their limits, making the effort to try to think what has not been thought before. We may allow ourselves to explore what provokes us and makes us uncomfortable and ask ourselves why it does so. And we may encourage larger jumps of associations, both when writing and reading, leaving behind the fear of not staying on topic, of not showing that we are clever and competent. Academic texts are now free to be less the result of the quasi-mechanical operations that are everywhere to be observed in academic journals, governed by editorial discipline. Texts can now be more the result of active choices of what we feel is needed and what we want.

2 So What Is Needed

What did I want to write? What did I perceive to be at stake, and feel that is needed? I want to emphasise the verb choice in the latter sentence: What did I *feel*? The question is not what a comprehensive literature review made me conclude about knowledge gaps or lacunae. The choice of the verb points inwards, towards the author subject. If no answer was to be found there, I might as well leave the writing to Microsoft Copilot.

This brings me to the question of my positioning. For more than three decades I have tried to do epistemological work mainly within two fields of science (and practice, in particular public policy), namely life sciences and environmental sciences.

My first field was that of biomedicine, specifically biochemistry and molecular biology. I have done philosophical critiques, epistemological reflections and ethical and policy analyses of biomedical research, gradually expanding to biotechnology, clinical medicine and also nutrition science. I have witnessed and lived with several waves of scientific and technological optimism in these fields since the Human Genome project and later the emergence of functional genomics, the -omics sciences in general, systems biology and the imaginaries and practices of precision medicine.

The other field that originally opened itself to me because of the epistemological and political complexities of the use of biotechnology in agriculture is that of environmental science and policy. I have become increasingly interested in and concerned by global environmental problems and what euphemistically is called sustainability challenges, such as climate change, soil erosion, water scarcity, pollution, biodiversity loss and habitat and ecosystem destruction.

At the core, both fields involve biology and its use in human decisions. Of course, there are immediate connections between the two fields that are evident to everybody, witnessed in the initiatives about "One Health", to take a prominent example. The focus of One Health has been to show how human health and the health of wild and domesticated animals are entangled into each other, especially when it comes to infections and epidemics. When animal populations are crowded and cramped, dangerous epidemics may intensify and endanger also our admittedly crowded and cramped human populations.

More than often, however, my research life devoted to the epistemology of biomedicine and environmental science has been an experience of living in two worlds and being plagued with the headaches of rampant cognitive dissonance. More than that, it has been an experience of *affective* and normative dissonance and a sense of discrepancy.

The sense of discrepancy is, of course, already a favourite substrate for (social) epistemological critique already within each of these two domains. Philosophers of science as well as STS scholars (and many others) have written lengthy analyses of the discrepancy e.g. between imaginaries and promises of precision medicine and what actually can be achieved if what we scientifically know about human biology, psychology and sociology is to be believed (Bremer & Strand, 2022). Equivalently, there are long-standing debates about what to believe about the state of affairs of natural environments and sustainability challenges. For example, some scientists and scholars see the prospects of a circular economy as the solution, while other scientists and scholars consider it a hype or even an expression of delirium (Giampietro, 2023). There is a whole literature that tries to describe, conceptualise and explain the phenomenon of discrepancy at the interface of science and public policy, employing concepts such as hypocognition (Giampietro & Funtowicz, 2020), social construction of ignorance (Rayner, 2012), and sociotechnical imaginaries (Jasanoff, 2019). I have discussed earlier how imaginaries may even take the flavour of becoming *fantasies* when they are proposed, maintained and performed in the presence of scientific knowledge that directly contradicts their content (Strand, 2022), and how the engagement into fantasies may develop into a form of escapism from the troubles of the real world (Strand, 2024).

Such expositions of discrepancy—that is, the experience that *others* display discrepancy—are valuable, I believe, and I have done my share of this kind of work. At the same time, they are a low-risk type of texts. One takes the position as the external critic who is criticising somebody else who should have known or done better. Towards the end of the piece, one might feel the need to say something constructive, to offer a way forward—either pushed by one's own internal sense of shame or duty, or by request from an unimpressed reviewer. At least when speaking for myself, I can confess that such "positive" or "constructive" endings have often tended to be quite short and feeble.

So, this is not what I will try to do here. Or will I? What else can such a text do?

Before discussing the possible end of this chapter, however, I will return to the key concept introduced above: What do I *feel* is needed? What do I feel, moving within and *between* these two worlds? Recalling that I do not have to be confined to displays of cleverness and competence, how do I want to describe the experience?[1] For example, how does it feel to spend one day at a precision medicine conference where bright scientists discuss the prospects of eradicating disease by knowing all genes in all detail and thereby tailoring medication and diet so that patients can have a super-long and super-healthy life, and then the next day sit in on meetings with environmental authorities and scientists who are concerned about impending ecological tipping points that, to use one catchphrase, might be incompatible with long-term or even short-term existence of the human species? How is it to listen one day to scientific prospects of precisely navigating individual health by lifestyle, food, drugs and of course apps, and the next day listen to scientific concerns about how global food security may well collapse because of the ongoing pollinator decline?

Answering without censorship: Sometimes when I move between these worlds I feel like I am losing my mind, that I am losing my sense of coherence in the world. Sometimes I find myself asking if I am going crazy, or if it is the world that has become crazy. I would like to cry out, but how? Turning to a jeremiad?

> I would comfort myself in sorrow;
> My heart is faint in me.
> Listen! The voice,

[1] An early-career colleague reminded me of how privileged I am who enjoy a permanent position as a professor at a state-owned public university in Northern Europe and can publish as I wish without jeopardising my job security. I hope the readers will read my claims about «no more need to be good boys and girls» as hopes and calls for change, rather than affirmative claims about empirical matters. Reality as of 2025 is of course stark for many early- and mid-career researchers, with political economies of «publish or perish» and academic cultures of discipline, repression and fear.

The cry of the daughter of my people
From a far country:
"Is not the Lord in Zion?
Is not her King in her?"
(Book of Jeremiah, 8:18–19)

What is needed, perhaps, to describe my experience, is hence not taking on the role of the philosopher interpreting the world or the scientist predicting it, but to invoke the persona of the prophet. It is to lament that the world is broken and urge action for its healing, although I do not know what the action should amount to, or indeed how active it should be.

3 A Jeremiad

Invoking the prophet? Really?? At this point, I can imagine how some readers are shaking their heads in disbelief, as many friends and colleagues have done over the years. "Roger, you are being dramatic, you are exaggerating. We have to look for opportunities and remain optimistic! We have to be *positive*!"

The way to be positive is, according to this sort of well-intended advice, typically to focus on some particular promising development. It is to remind oneself that antibiotics, cortisone and modern anaesthetics have improved millions of lives, regardless of the verdict on whether the overall venture of modern medicine in general has been a success (Le Fanu, 2014). It is to celebrate recent advances in nutrition science and consider current epidemics of, say, obesity or psychiatric eating disorders as external and irrelevant to that celebration. It is to applaud advances in wind and solar and other types of presumably "clean" energy production and not being thrown out of balance by the fact that not only global energy consumption but also global fossil fuel consumption and global carbon emissions increase every year so far, regardless of technological and political efforts to the contrary. To be positive is to *zoom in* and *stay on topic*, that is, stay talking about the part of the picture chosen for zooming in. To try to zoom out and invoke the Keeling curve in a discussion about wind and solar energy is, according to such well-meant advice, off topic, negative and unreasonable because it leads straight into defaitism, negativity and the belief that individual actors and actions are worthless to the big picture. That defaitism itself is not founded in evidence, the advice would go, and we should zoom in as there is no other way of solving big problems than developing piecemeal solutions.

From an epistemological perspective the storyline of such advice is highly interesting. It comes equipped with implicit reductionist theories of change (problems are solved step by step by zooming in, finding solutions at that level and scaling them up) that half imply normative positions both of an epistemological and ethical/political nature. The ethical or political position is the prescription of zooming in, since problems should be solved and this is the way to solve them. The implicit epistemological claim is that zooming in is the right way of looking at the world. Zooming out leads to confusion, to drifting off topic.

This type of storyline can be connected to reductionist thought at least back to René Descartes but also to what Rommetveit (Rommetveit et al., 2013) called the Bios discourse. By Bios he referred to a discourse that emerged in the twentieth century around a version of the grand narrative of Enlightenment and Modernity that took the successes of modern life science and biotechnology as its paradigm case and included economic growth as a main objective and success criterion.

According to Rommetveit, however, the development of Bios was accompanied by what he called the *Geos* discourse. Geos found its core not in life science but in the emerging system sciences of the environment (ecology, climate science, oceanography and earth science), which increasingly warned about limits to growth at the system level. Indeed, the concern for global environmental problems could only be stated scientifically by zooming out and trying to know the world at the macro scale, at the level of systems.

We have explained in previous work how the relationship between Bios and Geos is one of dissonance, and how this dissonance creates discrepancies in public policy (Kovacic et al., 2019). Global environmental problems need the Geos discourse to become visible and knowable, but it is hard to elaborate solutions from within this discourse, other than pragmatically quite empty statements such as "we have to cut emissions". Within the Geos discourse, one can think in terms of system states at the macro level and, essentially, the *outcomes* of actions. What is difficult within Geos is to ideate and imagine solutions. In practice, therefore, public policies try to translate problems defined in Geos, into problems that can be solved in Bios, by zooming in and employing reductionist methodologies to prescribe actions. All in all, this might be seen as contemporary modern societies' way of reflexive modernisation. Borrowing Ulrich Beck's terminology, it is acknowledged that we are living in a risk society in which modern technologies, institutions and practices produce and redistribute harms and risks as well as benefits. The responsible way of dealing with those harms and risks, however, according to what at least until early twenty-first century was considered mainstream politics in many countries in the Global North (as expressed and performed by "moderate" parties and major inter-and supranational organisations such as the OECD and the European Union) was to zoom in, stay on topic and stay positive. It was to engage in solutionism. It is no surprise that the Large Language Model chatbots reproduce this type of discourse; in the early twenty-first century, it is dominant.

The unsolved problem of sustainability governance, however, is that the outcomes of solutionist policies and actions very rarely matter in the big picture, at the system level. As a result, most global environmental problems are aggravating and escalating rather than residing, in spite of decades of political and public attention (European Environment Agency, 2024).

For environmental scientists—those I imagined sitting in with on the second day in the previous section—the discrepancy might appear to call for more power to environmental science. Rather than the jeremiad they might want more and louder (system) science advice, believing that radically more of the same advice finally is going to solve the problems. Geos should get louder. My problem—my positioning and my personal problem—is that I move between the two worlds of Bios and Geos, of life science and environmental science and their corresponding realms of governance and public policy—and cannot but agree that within each world there is rationality, there are good reasons and valid matters of care and concern. As one policymaker once told me, when confronted with critiques of economic growth: "So if we have population growth, and you don't want economic growth, tell me who should not eat then". Likewise, who is going to tell our population that knowledge, technology and policy aiming to tackle short-term population health and welfare issues are no longer valid enterprises? One Health is a nice idea and a legitimate concept, especially in the field of infectious medicine. And in a long-term helicopter perspective, zooming out, humanity has to stop its war and violence against other species. But here and now, there are painful contradictions and conflicts. Nature loss is caused by actions that try to respond to actual human needs. My personal problem is that I move between worlds, or bubbles if one wishes to call them so, in which the solution in one world may aggravate the problems in the other, and vice versa. One may dream of win-win solutions, but reality is more often than not that the problems are *wicked*, with small prospects of consensus on what is an acceptable solution (European Environment Agency, 2024).

Thus, *"I would comfort myself in sorrow; My heart is faint in me."*

And then, as I engage in lament and grief and allow comforting myself in sorrow, it occasionally feels easier afterwards to come to terms with reality—to accept that we are living in a wounded world (Haraway, 2016) and should expect to experience cognitive, affective and normative dissonance. From the persona of the prophet, it feels easier to return to the stance of the epistemologist, asking again: What can be known? Staying with the trouble, we can ask ourselves with renewed courage: What do we *know*, in contrast to what we *hope*?

4 Biopolitics and Acceleration

What do we know? A first observation is that even if I have been lamenting my moving between two worlds, there is only one world. Whether we consider it a world of multiple "bubbles", subsystems, discourses or "realities", at one level the world is one and whatever set of distinctions and divisions we prefer, they are not isolated from each other. One thing we know about this one world, is what I set out as the point of departure:

The Industrial Revolution laid the foundation for two dramatic changes in the human condition. It set off sociotechnical trajectories of exponential growth in human production and consumption in what has been called the Great Acceleration. On the one hand, this offered unprecedented technological capabilities at the individual and collective level. On the other, it led to unprecedented environmental problems and risks to the extent that sustainability science feared irreversible collapse of ecological and socio-ecological systems. Simultaneously, as part of these sociotechnical trajectories, a new form of politics arose by which it became a legitimate concern of the modern state to govern the size of its human population and the health state of its individual subjects. In this development of biopolitics and biopower, medicine, nutrition science and food science came to play important roles. With the very best intentions, these sciences have developed within a logic of control-and-command and with hopes of governing human populations towards long, healthy, productive and well-nourished lives.

The key passage in this statement is "simultaneously, as a part of these sociotechnical trajectories". Modern biopolitical states came to develop governance of population size and population health as a productive force in capitalist economies (as well as in socialist economies). A big, well-nourished and healthy population was and is spoken of as an end in itself, but fundamentally it is also a resource and a precondition for fast and growing production and consumption. A big and healthy population provides workers for industry, soldiers for wars, and consumers that sustain the circular flow of money and goods. The Great Acceleration of exponentially growing production and consumption rates, pollution and extraction of natural resources is a direct consequence of biopolitics. There is even almost a linear relationship across countries between indicators of human development and indicators of ecological footprint, with a handful of exceptions, such as Vietnam (European Environment Agency, 2024; O'Neill et al., 2018).

The scientific and political interest in nutrition was and still is at the heart of biopolitics. We can imagine that humans throughout the ages have developed knowledge about food and its role in health and well-being; and not only humans. There are also many precursors to modern nutrition science, for example early scientific interest in scurvy, beriberi and other deficiency diseases. Modern nutrition sciences and policies, however, emerged in the nineteenth and twentieth centuries, together with and within industrialisation and rapid population growth.

The scientific interest in macro-nutrients, while also a result of what we might call "basic research" in chemistry, found its societal relevance in the attempts at rationally planning and governing food supplies and food intakes for industrially organised populations such as factory workers and soldiers. In our time, we may see the same phenomenon not the least in national and international governance of populations of refugees and other displaced people. Calories and protein content are variables that are important when "seeing as a state" (Scott, 1998); individual obsession with these variables, as we find it in contemporary psychiatric eating disorders, is more to be seen as the unfortunate adoption of the scientific, biopolitical and objectifying gaze at the individual level, towards oneself.

We may ascribe this development to industrialisation (which I just did) or to capitalism (although it seems difficult to argue that socialist states were highly different). Hartmut Rosa has argued that there is a mechanism of alienation at an even deeper level in modern societies, which he calls "acceleration" (Rosa, 2019). At the macro-level, between states and economies, logics of competition and competitiveness accelerate economic activities because all actors have to fight for comparative advantage. For Rosa, however, continuous acceleration is also to be seen at the level of the human individual. In particular, Enlightenment opens up the modern subject to a sceptical attitude towards traditional authorities that dictated personal values and articulated one's meaning and purpose in life. The modern subject was set free to search for her or his own meaning and purpose. With the risk of simplifying Rosa's argument too much, this freedom—this recognition that existence precedes essence, to invoke Sartre—can lead to lifestyles and life orientations that are intrinsically alienating. One may not feel confident to know one's meaning and purpose in life (yet), and then in the meantime one engages in a project of maximising one's wealth and health so as to be well provided when one finally is able to know one's purpose. This modern subject is of course also an excellent consumer—she or he is more than willing to spend attention and money on goods and services that support and enhance health and well-being, comfort and beauty.

In this way, Rosa provides an appealing explanation to how the objectifying and alienating gaze of nutrition science could migrate so easily into affluent populations within (and outside) the Global North. God appearing to be dead (or at least not so relevant anymore), and vocations and idealist causes becoming uncertain and risky endeavours, what one safely could do, was to invest in personal care, preventive medicine, and health maximisation by tuning mind and body. One could do exercise, control one's food intake and attend to other lifestyle factors to aim for a long and healthy life. And in a modern world where science increasingly became considered the main source of epistemic authority, the answers to what a healthy life entails were to be found in the life sciences, in particular medicine and nutrition science [Ref Jasanoff bio book]. The answer to the question "Am I well?" was to be found in medical diagnostic practices. The answer to "What should I eat?" was to be found in nutrition science. Hence, the modern subject became a sort of entity (a mind?) that *has* a body that should be an object of (self-)governance. In this process, *food* is increasingly reframed as *nutrition*, as can be witnessed in any European or North American supermarket and its variety of products with macro-nutrient identities: protein bars, protein puddings, keto bars and fat free yogurts. Likewise, eating is reframed as individual acts of governance of the body rather than a matter of cultural practices, shared identities and values and, ultimately, meaning and purpose of life.

Claiming that these are things we know, I do not intend to say that nutritional concerns are illegitimate or inherently alienating, or that nutrition science or biopolitics are illegitimate endeavours. I am simply trying to stay with the trouble and answer the question about what we know. The answer I am providing from this line of thought is that problematic aspects of modernity, from the individual level of being alienated from one's own body and one's own culture, community and tradition, to the global level of the Great Acceleration and the risk of ecological tipping points, are intrinsically linked to industrialisation and biopolitics. Furthermore, the scientific and political focus on nutrition has played a key role in this development. What normative implications to draw from this insight, is another question that I will pursue in the next section.

5 Normative Implications and Conclusions

The extended abstract presented at the beginning of this chapter stated two open questions. I shall attend to them now. At this point, the reader is unlikely to be surprised to find that there will be few normative answers and more an attempt to stay with the question "what do we know?", letting "we" refer to the heterogeneous conglomerate of knowledge production that can be found in academia and around.

The first question was: "What sciences will be sorely needed in the post-growth era, after the Great Acceleration?"

The question can be seen as tendentious or at least taking a stance on a knowledge claim: It assumes that the Great Acceleration has to end, as was already assumed in the extended abstract presented in the introduction:

Moving into the second quarter of the twenty-first century, the anomalies and fractures in the modern world are increasingly visible. The Great Acceleration cannot continue much longer. The Earth is becoming full of us, our waste and our livestock as we pollute and deplete natural resources. Modern biopolitical orders are cracking up into violent, non-or post-humanitarian disorder, now also in the Global North.

Again, we know for a fact that different scientists and scholars take different positions on this matter. Some (though not many) believe that there are no planetary boundaries, that Planet Earth can deliver infinite amounts of natural resources, or that technological advances make it possible to substitute and replace natural resources that run out of supply with others, or produce renewable energy in quantities that it make it possible to recycle used resources to the extent that there is no more need for virgin materials. This position has existed in academia at least since the nineteenth century, when its proponents came under the label of Cornucopians. Others seem to believe in a Singularity, a point in time from which not only the economy is dematerialised but also human existence: That we somehow get immortal and immaterial by being uploaded into digital media and clouds, perhaps, as if digital technologies are not themselves material objects that require natural resources. Or they subscribe to what Kenneth Boulding called "cowboy economies" and are ready to leave Wasteland Earth and move on to conquer and colonise other planets, first of all Mars. It would take another book chapter to critically examine such positions. For now, I will move on to argue that we surely know that many scientists and scholars take other positions and find it highly unlikely that planetary boundaries are not relevant and that there are no limits to growth. For the sake of argument, we may accordingly limit ourselves to pursue that latter position as at least one possibility. Doing that, we can discuss from the premise that the Great Acceleration has to stop at some point, either because humans have been able to deliberately transform their production and consumption systems or because Nature itself acts, in the sense that climate and weather patterns change, freshwater becomes scarce and polluted, ecosystem services decline and disappear, and so on.

What we cannot know yet, is whether humanity already at the present, in the first part of the twenty-first century, has moved into a phase transition of the planet's climate system and biosphere, and if we already have passed tipping points. The genre of natural disaster movies typically depicts the apocalypse as an abrupt event that takes place within days or perhaps some weeks or months. What is difficult to know now is the extent to which growing regional and geopolitical conflicts are already caused by resource scarcity, climate change and failing ecosystem services. In the Middle East as well as Sahel and other dry parts of Africa, fertile land and water are clearly part of the issue. Ukraine, on the other hand, has always been important for food security. The currently rising geopolitical tensions in the Arctic cannot be seen as independent from concerns over energy security.

Accordingly, it may be that humanity already is in the middle of an involuntary transformation away from the Great Acceleration that is nothing like a nicely planned and smooth transition into lower consumption levels. In the Norwegian language there is a proverb that literally translates to "when the manger is empty, the horses bite each other". If this is in part what one currently can witness, one could expect a long period of increasing conflict, unrest and war as long as the biosphere (from the human perspective, in terms of what it can offer us of support) remains a wounded world. To employ recent jargon from the European political scene, we might be in a "permacrisis".

It is impossible to know what kind of science and knowledge will be needed in such a period or era of post-growth and post-acceleration. What would surprise me, though, is if the current intensity in supporting life science and highly sophisticated technologies to fine-tune individual health and longevity, will remain for long a public priority. It may of course exist within bubbles of wealthy elites, and these bubbles can be significant in themselves. For most countries in the world, however, precision medicine or precision nutrition and other scientific constituents of what we could call personalised biopolitics, are already irrelevant—imagine Ukraine or Russia choosing this as their main priority any time soon—and the present (2025) administration in the USA also seems to turn away from such research agendas. For countries and societies in which basic food, water and energy security is at stake, one can expect research agendas to become more basic, too.

At the same time, the bubble of life science and biopolitics is—as mentioned—not small in itself. Part of the Great Acceleration is the increase in the human population, which again definitely is a result of increased longevity, not the least because it is affluent people who by far consume the most and who by far live the longest. One can always hope, as did already Marquis de Condorcet when faced with Malthusian thoughts, that with increased wealth and increased scientific knowledge, humans will by themselves become so rational, unselfish and morally sophisticated as to not want to have too many children or live too long. It seems unlikely that it is contemporary life science that will bring about that moral sophistication, though. One can hope that the social sciences and humanities—sociology, anthropology, philosophy, history, and ethics—could support the *Bildung* processes needed. Indeed, some of us, such as the present author, invest our work life into that hope, even without much evidence that supports it.

And yet, perhaps one of the positive sides of the kind of life sciences that work so hard for saving the life and health of individuals (mostly the affluent ones in the Global North), is that they are symbols of care, of in the shape of a modern, utopian utilitarian humanism?

As all philosophers of care have pointed out, however, care is not innocent. When caring for something, one chooses (consciously or not) to care less or not care for something else. This leads me to my second question: "Which conceptualisations of food and the good life will humans need to flourish after the downfall of biopolitics of nutrition and health?"

At this point in the text, there should remain no doubt that I anticipate large fields of science, indeed those that are currently most prestigious, to become increasingly irrelevant as we move or are thrown out of the Great Acceleration. Still, I find it difficult to imagine a transformation where humanity discards all knowledge about micro-and macronutrients, especially as scarcity increases. The precision medicine imaginary might become discarded together with current extreme biopolitical projects such as those of Northern Europe, of welfare state-governed maximisation of health, longevity and QALYs—quality-adjusted life years. Basic questions about hunger and deficiencies are likely to stay, however. Or so I hope, because if they do not, humanity may have moved away from compassion and care for those who suffer.

Having left cleverness to chatbots, the goal of the exercise of writing this book chapter has been to articulate what I *feel,* based on my experience of doing epistemological work while moving between life science and environmental science and policy. The question I just stated, about conceptualisations of food and good life in a future that is highly uncertain if at all knowable, cannot be answered by verified knowledge. Instead, to close this chapter, I shall return to what I feel. I feel the desire and hope that the "post-apocalyptic future", the future after the downfall of the current civilisation, which is founded on unsustainable production and consumption systems, will be able to move forward and find compassion, care, beauty and human flourishing that is not based on maximisation of health and longevity. I hope that this will help them create a society that is not based on what Hartmut Rosa called acceleration. One way of imagining such a future, is to look back and around, outside the bubble of modern science, biopolitics and nutrition, into pre-modern and non-modern societies and cultures, and the many non-modern aspects of contemporary so-called modern people. It would be to return to questions of substantive meaning and purpose. It would be to rediscover, also scientifically, what food has meant to people, across cultures, as long as we know, as a basic, constitutive part of the good life together with others: family, friends, animals, communities.

Food culture studies definitely already exist, often as a critical correction to nutrition science, sometimes with a direct expression of a contrarian identity, such as the field of "fat studies" that wish to criticise and create an alternative to implicit (and explicit) dominant normativity in modern society and science that discriminates against those with higher body weight. What I desire and hope, is that in a post-apocalyptic future, food culture studies become an important science at the core of building new cultures and societies. In such a science, there would still be room for knowledge about micro-and macro-nutrients, but the focus would be elsewhere. The focus would lie on how the meaning and value of food and eating can be at the core of new sustainable production and consumption practices, practices that, to paraphrase Heidegger, embed, recall and respect the insight that whenever we pour a glass of wine or share a loaf of bread, both heaven and earth are invoked and implicated, through the water cycles, the nutrient cycles, the soil, plants, animals and our own labour. It would, if one accepts such a word, be a science that embeds and works from the premise of the sacredness of Mother Earth and its many ways of providing us with food, and the sacredness of human interaction.

Acknowledgements I am grateful for the support that the chatbot service Microsoft Copilot offered me, as a discussion partner, and also by concretely giving ideas for the abstract. Furthermore, I want to thank Francina Saiz for constructive suggestions and support in the preparation of this book chapter.

References

Bremer, A., & Strand, R. (2022). *Precision oncology and cancer biomarkers: Issues at stake and matters of concern.* Springer Nature.

Deleuze, G., & Guattari, F. (1994). *What is philosophy?* Verso.

European Environment Agency. (2024). *Governance in complexity: Sustainability governance under highly uncertain and complex conditions.* Publications Office of the European Union. https://data.europa.eu/doi/10.2800/597121

Giampietro, M. (2023). Reflections on the popularity of the circular bioeconomy concept: The ontological crisis of sustainability science. *Sustainability Science, 18*(2), 749–754. https://doi.org/10.1007/s11625-022-01267-z

Giampietro, M., & Funtowicz, S. O. (2020). From elite folk science to the policy legend of the circular economy. *Environmental Science & Policy, 109*, 64–72. https://doi.org/10.1016/j.envsci.2020.04.012

Haraway, D. J. (2016). *Staying with the trouble: Making kin in the Chthulucene*. Duke University Press.

Jasanoff, S. (2019). *Can science make sense of life?* (1st ed.). Polity.

Kovacic, Z., Strand, R., & Völker, T. (2019). The circular economy in Europe: Critical perspectives on policies and imaginaries.

Le Fanu, J. (2014). *Rise and fall of modern medicine*. Abacus Software.

O'Neill, D. W., Fanning, A. L., Lamb, W. F., & Steinberger, J. K. (2018). A good life for all within planetary boundaries. *Nature Sustainability, 1*(2), 2. https://doi.org/10.1038/s41893-018-0021-4

Rayner, S. (2012). Uncomfortable knowledge: The social construction of ignorance in science and environmental policy discourses. *Economy and Society, 41*(1), 107–125. https://doi.org/10.1080/03085147.2011.637335

Rommetveit, K., Strand, R., Fjelland, R., Funtowicz, S., & Saltelli, A. (2013). *What can history teach us about the prospects of a European research area*. European Commission Joint Research Centre.

Rosa, H. (2019). *Resonance: A sociology of our relationship to the world*. Polity.

Scott, J. C. (1998). *Seeing like a state: How certain schemes to improve the human condition have failed*. Yale University Press.

Strand, R. (2022). The impact of a fantasy. In I. C. Beneduce & M. Bertolaso (Eds.), *Personalized medicine in the making: Philosophical perspectives from biology to healthcare* (pp. 311–324). Springer International Publishing. https://doi.org/10.1007/978-3-030-74804-3_16

Strand, R. (2024). Beyond Digital Escapism. In A. Fabris & S. Belardinelli (Eds.), *Digital environments and human relations: Ethical perspectives on AI issues* (p. 169–185). Springer Nature Switzerland. https://doi.org/10.1007/978-3-031-76961-0_9

The Complexity of Food Health Related Choices

Mario Giampietro and Sandra G. F. Bukkens

1 Introduction

In recent years the interest of consumers in the quality of food products has grown considerably, especially in developed societies (Kasriel-Alexander, 2016; Li & Kallas, 2021). This increased attention has focused on 'sustainable' alternatives to conventional techniques of food production, such as organic food (Canavari & Olson, 2007; IFOAM Organics Europe, 2023; Stolz et al., 2011; Yussefi-Menzler, 2010), alternative methods of food distribution (local production or zero-km-products) (DuPuis & Goodman, 2005; Martinez et al., 2010; Morgan, 2010; Murdoch et al., 2000; Mustapa & Kallas, 2025) and fair trade (Codron et al., 2006), as well as on human health and nutrition (e.g., functional foods (Sgroi et al., 2024)). Hence, the growing change in consumer attitude reflects a more general concern about the poor health

M. Giampietro (✉) · S. G. F. Bukkens
European Centre for Governance in Complexity (ECGC), Bergen, Norway
e-mail: mario.giampietro1@gmail.com

Universidad Científica del Sur, Lima, Peru

F. Bruno et al. (eds.), *Healthcare and Food*,
https://doi.org/10.1007/978-981-95-5899-5_3

(performance) of the existing structure and operation of the modern food system (Blay-Palmer 2016; Porter & Kramer, 2011).

However, in practice, the definition and analysis of food system health or performance and quality of food products have resulted in being elusive concepts. The relations between food system activities, human health, the environment, the economy and the cultural identity of a given society are extremely complex and impossible to represent in terms of a finite set of attributes that can be measured and modeled (Curvelo et al. 2019; Ericksen, 2008; Giampietro, 2004; Lang & Barling, 2012; McMichael, 2000; Sobal et al., 1998; Sonnino & Marsden, 2006; Tandon et al., 2020; Tansey G. & Rajotte, 2008; Tilman & Clark, 2014; Vorley, 2003). The more so as the globalization of the food system has become almost inevitable. Even in local production systems, most inputs, such as energy, fertilizer and animal feed, are imported and hence some of the impacts of the production system are externalized to distant ecosystems and societies (Billen et al., 2014; Cadillo-Benalcazar et al., 2020; Harder et al., 2021; Wang et al., 2022). Indeed, in dealing with complex issues, such as the production and consumption of food in a modern urban society, it is simply impossible to identify a set of attributes that can result in a substantive ranking of what is the 'best' (or the 'optimal') choice to make.

The term 'food credence attribute' has been put forward to indicate that most of the 'qualities' of a food product cannot possibly be properly evaluated by the consumer (Schrobback et al., 2023). This includes the impact of the food system (production, distribution and consumption of food products) on the environment, such as GHG emissions, impact on soil, water and biodiversity, as well as the impact on animal welfare, farmers' welfare and human health. Indeed, more often than not, consumers have to rely on trusted cues and information to assist them in assessing the food quality and credence attributes they seek at the point of purchase (e.g., nutritional information, organic production, animal welfare, zero-km-products, fair trade) (Wu et al., 2021). Producers, processors and retailers provide consumers with food safety and quality assurances, while government agencies, third-party institutions, advocacy groups, and the mass media may modify how labeling information and food operators are perceived by consumers (Laursen & Noe, 2017;

Wu et al., 2021). This situation makes food choices extremely complex due to (sometimes purposeful) lack of robust information and possible manipulation of consumer perceptions through marketing, government awareness programs and NGO action campaigns.

Furthermore, several studies on consumer attitude have shown that the definition of quality of a food product reflects not only the information available but also the normative values of the consumer (Gallie, 1994; Giampietro & Bukkens, 2015; Paloviita, 2010; Vivero-Pol, 2017). For this reason, there is also an unavoidable ethical dimension to any food choice, especially related to sustainability (the sustainability of our body, our family, our community, our natural environment, and climate change and global issues in general) (Andorfer & Liebe, 2013; Kjærnes, 2012; Manyukhina, 2017).

Hence, any quantitative analysis aimed at assessing the 'performance' of food systems faces an epistemological challenge that is common to all purposive quantitative analyses attempting to assess the performance of complex systems (Barnhill & Bonotti, 2023; Giampietro et al., 2006). Indeed, the problem faced by the scientist in generating an integrated assessment of the food system is similar to that faced by the consumer when purchasing food at the retailer, that is, the problem of 'simplification' of complexity. Simplifying an enormous information space into a simple protocol for selecting and ranking food items unavoidably generates hypocognition, i.e., the negligence of relevant aspects of the complex system under analysis due to their exclusion from the chosen analytical frame (Lakoff, 2010).

In the following section, we will illustrate the general problems faced when trying to characterize the performance of the modern food system and the resulting quality of its food products. We will show that these problems are rooted in the coexistence of many different dimensions and scales of analysis that must be considered and represented simultaneously according to the many non-equivalent perceptions and normative values of the various social actors involved. Then, we will frame this discussion in more technical terms: What are the problems faced when using multi-criteria analysis to rank options when dealing with complex food choices? Last but not least, we will argue that (i) moral choices must play a key role in the redefinition of a more sustainable food system, and (ii) that food should not be considered a mere commodity, but something special associated with the definition of our very identity.

2 The Complexity of Food Health Related Choices

The analysis of food choices in ecological systems is called foraging theory (Stephens & Krebs, 1986). Foraging theory studies how animals (including humans) make decisions about acquiring food and balancing the benefits of different food sources with associated costs and risks (Giraldeau, 2010). This definition indicates that for any animal in any ecological system, the nutritional quality of a food product is not the only attribute determining the convenience of its consumption; other factors are relevant in foraging choices, such as the energy cost of exploitation of the food resource, the time required, potential risks associated with the choice (e.g., predators), and negative consequences that the gathering and consumption of a particular food item may imply on other functions expressed by the foraging system. Hence, when assessing the performance of a foraging strategy, it is necessary to consider not only the phase of consumption of food items, but also the various processes required to make the food available to the final consumer.

In human beings, food choices are further complicated by moral and ethical aspects (conscious choices) (Andorfer & Liebe, 2013; Kjærnes, 2012; Manyukhina, 2017). Indeed, our perception of the quality of food products depends on a mix of factors:

1. The set of *positive attributes* that determines our food choice. These can be *direct* positive attributes, such as personal preferences, emotions and sensory appeal (in matters of taste, texture, brand, price, packaging, convenience, nutritional value) and *indirect* positive attributes such as social norms and cultural traditions (e.g., special or traditional foods eaten on special occasions).
2. The set of concerns associated with the production and consumption of food products and defining *negative attributes* of food products. Examples are concerns about the effect their consumption may have

on our health (e.g., pesticide residues, potential harmful food additives, high sugar or saturated fat content), our environment (nitrogen leakage, pesticide pollution, erosion of biodiversity, energy consumption), animal welfare, the local economy and distant countries/ecosystems (considering the consequences of imports).

3. The relative importance (weight) we give to our preferences and concerns when integrating these different pieces of information at the moment of deciding.

Hence, the analysis of the consequences of our food choices depends on personal, direct perceptions and on the knowledge claims we have available (what we know) about the direct and indirect effects of production and consumption of food. The process of decision-making related to food choices is thus necessarily complex (even for animals that do not have the complication of social and moral values) as it requires gathering and processing information in relation to:

1. *Criteria* relevant for characterizing the performance (food health) of a given choice. The relevance of these criteria is given by individual preferences (direct positive or negative attributes) and by societal concerns transmitted to the individual (indirect positive or negative attributes). These criteria can be derived from the justification narratives (normative beliefs) that inform our decision process, i.e., *why* we chose a given product.
2. *Indicators* needed for characterizing the performance of the choice in relation to the selected attributes. These indicators are determined by the endorsement of explanation narratives used to inform the decision process, i.e., *what* are the consequences and concerns associated with the choice of a given product. They reflect the existence of trust in existing knowledge claims about the expected attributes of performance of the chosen products.

Having said so, the third and last step is to analyze the process through which we make our decisions when considering the relative importance of relevant attributes and the pertinence and robustness of knowledge claims. Such an integrated assessment can be subject to large levels of uncertainty. How do we know that we are not neglecting important concerns? How do we know that the information we use to assess the implications of the consumption of a given food product (the knowledge claim) is reliable?

3. *Procedures* establishing priorities over the relevance of the indicators linked to the different criteria. Procedural choices are needed to handle the heterogeneous information space created by considering both criteria and indicators (each loaded with uncertainty) in individuating the "right" choice among all those possible, i.e., *how* to integrate normative and descriptive information about the consequences of food choices. A procedural choice has to compromise between justification narratives derived from individual preferences (direct positive attributes) and those derived from the social norms and values in the society in which the individual is operating (the concerns existing in society about the negative consequences—indirect negative attributes—and the beneficial effects of food choice—indirect positive attributes). This tension must be handled using available knowledge claims (epistemic beliefs) describing the consequences of the choice in relation to the relevant criteria of performance. Given that different individuals handle this tension in different ways, it is unavoidable to find, in any given society, the coexistence of legitimate but contrasting points of view and perspectives regarding food choices.

The above process of food health related choices of individual consumers is summarized in general terms in Fig. 1. As can be seen from Fig. 1, this process is in principle no different from the process of decision-making regarding other sustainability issues. Decision-making on sustainability problems always requires considering and weighting indicators referring to direct and indirect criteria of performance and handling a high level of uncertainty in knowledge claims while integrating legitimate but contrasting perspectives about what is "the best thing to do." Hence, in the next section we will use theoretical concepts and practical tools from the field of science for governance (i.e., decision

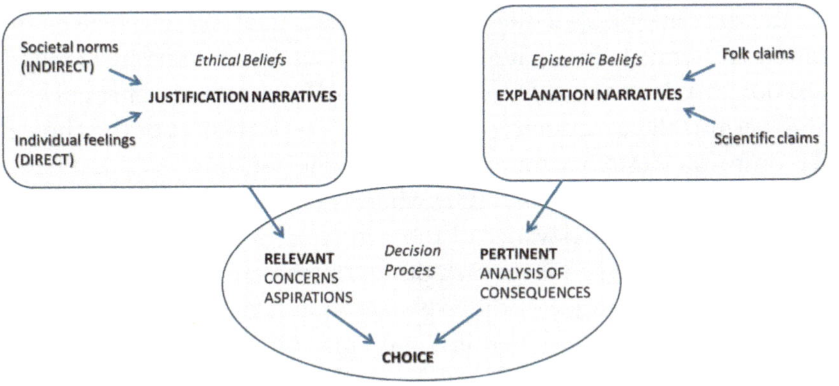

Fig. 1 The process determining food choices

theory) to further illustrate the predicament faced by consumers at the moment of making their food choices.

3 The Consumer's Predicament of Making Food Health Related Choices

Consider a consumer wanting to make food choices that contribute to the sustainability of the planet and that in society are generally believed to be desirable. To make a food choice fulfilling this purpose a 'responsible' consumer will need value-driven motivation for action (justification narratives) associated with ethical beliefs. Then, to translate these beliefs into action, the justification narratives must be associated with explanation narratives that allow a definition of the *desirable* state of affairs in relation to the choice to be made.

For example, if the state of affairs A is desirable (e.g., happy and healthy farm animals), whereas state of affairs B is undesirable (e.g., intensive livestock production), then there is a goal associated with the food choice that can be used to guide actions, i.e., move toward the state of affairs A (e.g., become vegetarian or purchase animal-welfare certified products). In this case, the explanation narrative should be able to describe the relevant attributes of this change (*what* should be changed) and causal relations (*how* the change will be beneficial) and hence represent an epistemic belief that allows the consumer to individuate a useful behavior in relation to the desired goal to be achieved. This epistemic belief permits the consumer to imagine the consequences of the choice in relation to the desired state of affairs (i.e., the consumer's ethical beliefs) (e.g., choice X entails A as result, whereas choice Y entails B as result). In this situation, the relevance of the two types of narratives (ethical and epistemic beliefs) depends on each other: the relevance of the justification determines the relevance of the explanation and vice versa.

In theory, by combining ethical and epistemic beliefs, the responsible consumer should be able to identify specific choices as 'right' or 'wrong.' However, in real life things are not that simple. Indeed, more often than not we find:

1. Non-equivalent narratives about causality co-exist. For example, one explanation narrative may say choice X leads to A (in relation to certain attributes) whereas another explanation narrative may say choice Y leads to A and/or choice X leads to B (when considering other attributes). This is called, in decision theory, *technical incommensurability*.
2. Several contrasting but legitimate perceptions of the desirability of the state of affairs co-exist. For example, some may perceive B as bad and A as good, whereas others perceive B as good and A as bad. This is called, in decision theory, *social incommensurability*.

In such a situation, the decision-making (choice) of the responsible consumer becomes difficult. What if the consumer has no clear perception of the desirability of the state of affairs at all? What if the consumer has a clear picture but that picture is not shared by others in her/his social circle? What if the presumed cause–effect relation between choice and consequences is incorrect? What if the relation between cause and effect simply cannot be known? In practice, good intentions of responsible consumers do not necessarily guarantee that 'the right choice' in relation to their ethical beliefs will be made.

Examples of the uncertainty inherent in epistemic beliefs are abundant for ethical beliefs (justification narratives) aimed at "saving the world," i.e., reducing climate change, saving the natural environment, ending animal suffering. For instance, the ethical belief that humans must reduce their impact on the biosphere is often translated, using explanation narratives, into a vision that people should contribute to this mission (desirable state of the food system) by avoiding the consumption of meat and fish (vegetarianism) or avoiding the consumption of all products of animal origin (veganism). However, depending on the scale at which the explanation narrative is applied we may have different technical assessments about the effect of these choices.

The explanation narrative related to the short time scale, usually is that by not eating meat and other animal products (e.g., milk, eggs), we discourage intensive livestock production and in this way reduce (or avoid altogether) the double conversion of feed crops (such as grains) into meat, thus making more grains available for direct consumption and reducing the need for arable land. In this narrative, meat consumption is perceived as undesirable given that a diet rich in meat implies grain production and consumption per capita that is three times that of a vegetarian diet. Reducing meat consumption reduces the need for crop production, allowing the possibility of restoring terrestrial ecosystems.

However, in the long term, a vegetarian diet may enhance an increase in population density as by avoiding the double conversion of crops into meat it will become possible to feed more people with a given area of land. In support of this argument, consider China whose population has historically had a relatively low meat consumption. China has approximately the same land area as the USA but almost four times more people inhabiting the land. Also note that well before the industrial revolution and the resulting explosion in the population size, a diet rich in meat was adopted during the course of human evolution in all regions with fragile ecosystems (e.g., pastoralists in semi-desertic areas and in arctic areas) because pastoralism forces respect for the environment (i.e., the entire set of relations in the trophic chains of local ecosystems). On the contrary, vegetarian diets consist mostly of only a limited number of selected plant species (grains, tubers), the monocultures of which tend to dramatically reduce biodiversity in terrestrial ecosystems.

In the case of animal-welfare certified products, the uncertainty also concerns the question of for whom the choice is beneficial. While the choice may be beneficial for the cow, it may not be for the welfare and well-being of the animal farmer because of an increase in production costs (Appleby, 2005; Kato et al., 2024). Animal-welfare certification may increase the price of meat and meat products for the consumer, and if no alternatives are available, this may affect the option to purchase meat and animal products for the lower-income classes (Appleby, 2005; Lusk, 2011; Lusk & Norwood, 2011; Olsen et al., 2024).

These examples show that even if we have a valid motivation for action (the justification narrative of lowering the environmental impact), the consequence of the food choice made to achieve the goal will depend on the robustness of the epistemic beliefs associated with the explanation narrative about cause and effect and the priority given to short-term versus long-term considerations and to the different actors in the food system. Accepting the coexistence of different explanation narratives about causal relations (epistemic beliefs) referring to the same value-driven motivations for action (ethical beliefs or justification narratives) entails acknowledging that for individual consumers it is challenging to obtain a robust analysis and a shared perception of priorities in relation to a given time span.

4 The Analyst's Predicament of Analyzing Food Health Related Choices

Societal Multi-Criteria Analysis

Any analyst faces a similar problem to that of the consumer when it comes to assessing the performance (health) of food production and consumption. In line with the considerations in the previous sections, Checkland (1999) and Checkland and Scholes (1990) have argued that for any 'messy reality' involving a virtually unlimited number of perspectives, goals, narratives and relevant attributes, the most important steps of any integrated assessment are the choices made in the pre-analytical phase. It is in the compression of the virtually infinite information space into the finite amount of information used to make the choice, that the analyst must repeatedly ask her/himself whether she/he is performing a heroic compression or brutal and terrible simplification (Reinert, 2007; Saltelli et al., 2020). Especially on the normative side, the compression of information often implies a selective filtering of values that reflects the existence of asymmetries in power relations. In this regard, several authors have proposed an iterative process of compressing, re-expanding, re-compressing (Röling & Wagemakers, 1998; Stirling, 2003).

Indeed, it is for a good reason that instead of the term 'multi-criteria analysis' (a term associated with the idea of a formal output) the term 'societal multi-criteria evaluation' (a term associated with the idea of a process) has been proposed (Munda, 2004; Munda, 2008). In societal multi-criteria evaluation, the problem structuring is based on reaching an agreement on:

1. the set of different relevant attributes (referring to different criteria of performance) that have to be considered simultaneously,
2. the set of indicators to characterize the performance in relation to the chosen set of attributes,
3. the procedures to be used for handling the different pieces of information derived from the selected (non-equivalent) indicators defined at different scales and dimensions.

To further illustrate the importance of the procedure of problem structuring, we use an example of an integrated assessment of a change (a presumed improvement) in the technical process of milk production proposed by a private company. According to conventional economic assessments (i.e., cost benefit analysis) of the performance of technologies, any reduction in production costs obtained by an increased efficiency and/or productivity should be perceived as an 'improvement.' The underlying ethical justification of such narrative is the utilitarian tradition, which is based on the principle of generating the maximum benefit for the maximum number of people (Bentham, 1907; Mill, 1879). By adopting this economic narrative, we can readily calculate a simple quantitative index of productivity (e.g., a given rate of milk flow per cow per day) that is linked to economic performance. For instance, the daily net milk produced per cow (yearly average) was less than 5 liters in preindustrial farms, whereas it can reach up to 30 liters in modern 'milk factories' (USDA-NASS 2025). In this line of thought, actions that enable to produce more useful products at a lower cost are 'good' and the most efficient process of milk production is "the best." Accepting this definition of a desirable state of affairs and the associated narrative, science-driven innovations in milk production are good since they have led to impressive improvements in efficiency. But is this numerical index of efficiency effective in defining whether or not we are witnessing a genuine improvement? Is 'more' or 'cheaper' necessarily better? Better for whom? Under which assumptions should we consider an increase in productivity or efficiency in a production system an improvement?

Indeed, a higher production rate and/or greater efficiency can be considered a true improvement only under the ceteris paribus clause; that is, "all other things remaining the same" (the essence of reductionism). In real life, this is never the case for important technological changes. In the case of milk production there may be changes in farm infrastructure, well-being of the farmer, well-being of the cows, resource use per liter of milk, environmental impact, milk quality (nutritional composition, contaminants) and/or final consumer price. But then which, if any, of these side effects should be included in the assessment? How reasonable is it to assume that a liter of milk remains 'the same' regardless of the nature of the production process? That is not to say that an increased productivity/efficiency is necessarily "bad," but that the characterization of changes in the performance of agricultural systems should be done carefully, using an integrated set of indicators that allows better understanding the pros and cons of the changes proposed. A richer description is needed, considering the diverse aspects of milk production and the perceptions of all social actors affected/involved. This will require a larger set of criteria of performance (what are the relevant attributes to be considered in the analysis?) and related indicators and targets (associated with desirable states of affairs). In other words, it is essential to contextualize the indications given by any single numerical index of performance by integrating this information with other indicators of performance referring to different perceptions of the desirability of the state of affairs. The perception of a 'problem' (or concern) results from a discrepancy between the desired state (what is expected), defined in normative terms (ethical beliefs) by "a storyteller" and the perceived state (what is experienced), defined in descriptive terms (epistemic beliefs) by "that storyteller."

Popular tools for organizing the information space used to make a choice in multi-criteria analysis (Munda, 2008) are:

1. The impact matrix, which is related to the chosen *epistemic* beliefs. The impact matrix covers the epistemological aspects of the assessment, that is, how to describe the current state of affairs and make anticipatory models of the consequences of our choices (using explanation narratives).
2. The equity matrix, which concerns the chosen ethical beliefs. The equity matrix covers ethical aspects of the assessment: how to reflect on the consequences of different value-driven motivations for action (justification narratives). For instance, the generation of winners and losers among the different actors carrying contrasting ethical beliefs.

The Impasses Linked to the Use of the Impact Matrix and the Equity Matrix

The Impact Matrix (Descriptive Side)

To transform a chosen attribute (referring to only one of the relevant characteristics to be observed) into an operational indicator, we have to define a range of values for the selected proxy variable associated with the performance, that is acceptable and/or desirable (target values). In this way, we can assess the expected performance of the choice in relation to this target. For example, with regard to animal welfare, we need a series of proxy variables (health aspects, space available, time spent outside grazing, life expectancy) to assess the performance in relation to the criterion animal welfare. For instance, a target informing the evaluation could be "the life expectancy of a cow must be at least 15 years" rather than the five years typical of cows producing large quantities of milk per day.

In Fig. 2, a simplified example of an impact matrix is shown, which shows a multi-criteria representation of the performance of various alternative processes used for supplying milk. The categorization of attributes is based on disciplinary knowledge. The use of this matrix assumes that the selected set of indicators (not shown in Fig. 2) as well as the target for each indicator (not shown in Fig. 2 but determining the "color" of the assessment) are expected to be relevant and have been agreed upon by all social actors involved and affected by the choice (something that is extremely unlikely in real cases). Whether or not the target is reached by a given process is indicated in Fig. 2 by the green (target achieved), yellow (sometimes achieved sometimes not) and red (target not achieved) symbols. More elaborated examples of impact matrices are available in the literature (e.g., (Feliciano et al., 2024; Hellstrand, 2006; Springmann, 2024)).

The representation given by an impact matrix typically illustrates the problem of technical incommensurability. Technical incommensurability refers to the impossibility of integrating the information derived from different explanation narratives that are based on non-equivalent

Dimensional criteria	*relevant attributes*	High Tech Production	Organic Production	Subsistence Production
Economic	Added value	✓	✓	✗
	Rural Development	✗	✓	✗
Consumer health	Milk Quality	✓	✓ ✓	!
	Safety	✓	✓	✗ ✗
Food security	Reliable supply	✓	✓	!
	Convenience	✓	!	✗
Environmental Health	GHG-emissions	✗	!	✓
	NP-leakages	✗	✓	✓
	Loss of habitat	✗	✗	✓
Cow welfare	Life expectancy Grazing	✗	✓	✓ ✓

Fig. 2 Example of an impact matrix for different milk production systems

descriptive domains with different scales (e.g., cow, farm, rural area, or consumer, society) and dimensions (economic, health, ecological, etc.) at which the operations of the food system and the implications of our choices are perceived and represented.

The Equity Matrix (Normative Side)

In Fig. 3, we illustrate a simplified (and hypothetical) equity matrix characterizing the effects of different government regulations (e.g., U.S. Farm Bills) on different agents operating in the dairy system. In this matrix we consider the relevance given to the selected attributes by different storytellers.

The rows represent the various social actors and stakeholders involved in or affected by the choice of regulation, the columns the various possible regulations considered in the information and decision space. To construct this matrix, participatory processes are required in which social actors are asked for their opinions (their specific personal choices) about

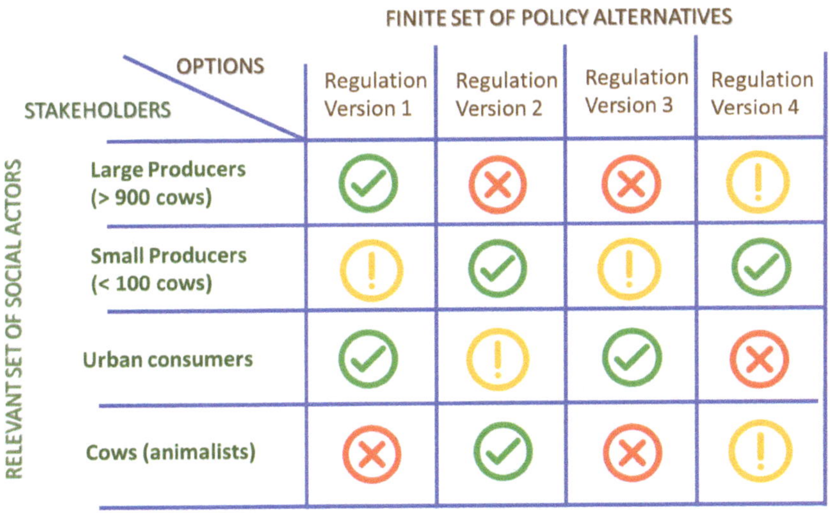

Fig. 3 Example of an equity matrix characterizing the perceptions of the effects of different government regulations of different agents operating in the dairy system

a given set of regulations or policy options. Their feedback is an 'overall' reaction on the various dimensions of milk production (see Fig. 2), in which reasoning, common sense and emotions all play a role.

The equity matrix is highly relevant for analyzing:

1. Power relations and conflicts. In the case of a specific decision, the equity matrix clearly shows the winners and the losers. Hence, in the case of conflicting choices it is useful to study the potential of the formation of coalitions.
2. The adequacy of chosen narratives, criteria and indicators. The equity matrix offers the opportunity to ask the various social actors about the narratives, criteria and indicators that determine their opinion and final choice. This may reveal the existence of important narratives that were neglected in the initial formulation of the problem structuring.
3. The adequacy of the given option space. The social actors can also provide an evaluation of the set of options considered (the various regulations) and suggestions for alternative options. Indeed, in a participatory integrated assessment, new policy options may emerge as a result of the negotiation among social actors.

In conclusion, the equity matrix illustrates the effects of social incommensurability as well as the policy implications of the coexistence of different legitimate perspectives about the "best choice." The social incommensurability is generated by differences in: (i) the prioritization of justification narratives, which relates to the different aspirations, moral values, fears and taboos of different storytellers; (ii) the heterogeneity of the available knowledge claims for creating the information space used to make a (final) choice.

For further examples of social multi-criteria analysis and impact and equity matrices, see, for example, (Ashofteh et al., 2017; Giampietro & Bukkens, 2015; Mazzetto & Bonera, 2003; Munda, 2008; Scuderi & Sturiale, 2016; Sjöström et al., 2019).

5 Post-Normal Science: Procedural Choices under Uncertainty

In the field of science for governance, post-normal science has been proposed to handle scientific inquiry and decision-making when dealing with complex issues, "where facts are uncertain, values in dispute, stakes high and decisions urgent" (Funtowicz & Ravetz, 1993; Funtowicz & Ravetz, 1990b; Funtowicz & Ravetz, 1990a). The main purpose of post-normal science is guaranteeing the quality of the process of decision-making when it involves both social and technical incommensurability (S. O. Funtowicz & Ravetz, 1994; S. Funtowicz & Ravetz, 1990a). Given the nature of the problems associated with the food choices of individual consumers, and the analysis of food production systems by analysts, the theory and practices required by post-normal science are particularly useful in this field.

Applying the idea of post-normal science to food health related choices, we see that a procedural choice must guarantee three quality criteria in the process of decision-making (see Fig. 1):

1. On the normative side, the procedure requires a check on the quality and usefulness of the problem structuring in relation to the knowledge claims selected and used. Is the proposed problem structuring adequate for the selection of relevant entities and options to be implemented? Who decided how to establish the inclusion and exclusion of justification narratives and the priorities over contrasting justification narratives? Who decided the options (e.g., the various production systems) considered in the analysis and why were only those considered relevant?
2. On the descriptive side, the procedure requires a check on the quality and usefulness of the representation given by the integrated analysis (the information provided by the impact matrix in Fig. 2). Is the proposed representation plausible and useful for deliberation? Is the given quantitative representation pertinent and correct according to verified knowledge claims? Can the selected attributes perhaps be better characterized with other observables, other models, other indicators? Regarding the plausibility of the results, are we checking

narratives that are addressing both the steady-state view (short-term view—ceteris paribus) and the evolutionary view (long-term view—"*ceteris are never paribus*")?

3. On the process of decision-making itself (reflexivity), the procedure requires a check on: (i) the selection and prioritization of the justification narratives used to define the relative importance of the attributes considered at the moment of the choice; (ii) the quality and effectiveness of the process used to validate the knowledge claims; and (iii) the mechanism used to weight the consequences of the choice against the relative priority over the different concerns. This process of weighting has nothing to do with scientific reasoning. Indeed, it is simply impossible to define 'the best' or 'optimal' solution for a given problem structuring without having first reached an agreement on the set of relevant criteria, the robustness of the quantitative analysis and the relative priority assigned to the different justification narratives.

6 Conclusions

This chapter has explored the complexity of food health related choices and has shown that in this field we find an example of a more generalized problem encountered in the decision-making process of complex and wicked issues. The main points to drive home are:

1. When dealing with choices involving the environmental health of food production (sustainability), the attributes used for the decision are always credence attributes, no matter what choice has to be made.
2. When dealing with complex issues, such as the production and consumption of food, it is impossible to identify a set of attributes and frame a multi-criteria analysis that is capable of generating a substantive ranking indicating the "best" or "optimal" choice.
3. An unavoidable ethical dimension is faced in any choice associated with food health (the sustainability of our body, our family, our landscape, our community, the entire society). The complexity of the

issue entails an unavoidable level of uncertainty about the future consequences of all food choices.

Individual consumers eager to improve food health with their food choices face a mission impossible. As they are unable to assess the full consequences of their choices, they cannot rely on an ethical consequentialism stand, nor can they assume by default that their beliefs are absolutely true and therefore their choices cannot rely on an ethical deontological stand. The issue is far too complex for adopting either of these two solutions. Given that large doses of uncertainty are associated with their decision process, the only option left is "to do what seems appropriate" rather than "the best thing." This is a reformulated (softened) version of the virtue ethics stand. Individual human beings—in contrast to scientific analysts—deal with this moral dilemma without going through a fair and democratic process of deliberation. They are led by emotions (moods) and can only consult their conscience before choosing, even when the decision is urgent and the uncertainty high.

References

Andorfer, V. A., & Liebe, U. (2013). Consumer behavior in moral markets. On the relevance of identity, justice beliefs, social norms, status, and Trust in Ethical Consumption. *European Sociological Review, 29*(6), 1251–1265. https://doi.org/10.1093/ESR/JCT014

Appleby, M. C. (2005). The relationship between food prices and animal welfare. *Journal of Animal Science, 83*(suppl_13), E9–E12. https://doi.org/10.2527/2005.8313_supplE9x

Ashofteh, P.-S., Bozorg-Haddad, O., & Loáiciga, H. A. (2017). Multi-criteria environmental impact assessment of alternative irrigation networks with an adopted matrix-based method. *Water Resources Management, 31*(3), 903–928. https://doi.org/10.1007/s11269-016-1554-9

Barnhill, A., & Bonotti, M. (2023). Healthy eating policy and public reason in a complex world: Normative and empirical issues. *Food Ethics, 8*(2), 1–19. https://doi.org/10.1007/S41055-023-00131-9/METRICS

Bentham, J. (1907). *An Introduction to the Principles of Morals and Legislation.* Clarendon Press. https://oll.libertyfund.org/titles/bentham-an-introduction-to-the-principles-of-morals-and-legislation

Billen, G., Lassaletta, L., & Garnier, J. (2014). A biogeochemical view of the global agro-food system: Nitrogen flows associated with protein production, consumption and trade. *Global Food Security, 3*(3–4), 209–219. https://doi.org/10.1016/j.gfs.2014.08.003

Blay-Palmer, A. (2016). *Food fears: From industrial to sustainable food systems* (1st ed.). Routledge. https://doi.org/10.4324/9781315582658

Cadillo-Benalcazar, J. J., Renner, A., & Giampietro, M. (2020). A multiscale integrated analysis of the factors characterizing the sustainability of food systems in Europe. *Journal of Environmental Management, 271*, 110944. https://doi.org/10.1016/j.jenvman.2020.110944

Canavari, M., & Olson, K. D. (2007). Organic food. Consumers' choices and farmers' opportunities. In M. Canavari & K. D. Olson (Eds.), *Organic food. Consumers' choices and farmers' opportunities*. Springer. https://doi.org/10.1007/978-0-387-39582-1

Checkland, P. (1999). *Systems thinking, systems practice: Includes a 30-year retrospective*. Wiley.

Checkland, P., & Scholes, J. (1990). *Soft-systems methodology in action.* John Wiley.

Codron, J. M., Siriex, L., & Reardon, T. (2006). Social and environmental attributes of food products in an emerging mass market: Challenges of signaling and consumer perception, with European illustrations. *Agriculture and Human Values, 23*(3), 283–297. https://doi.org/10.1007/S10460-006-9000-X/METRICS

Curvelo, I. C. G., Watanabe, E. A. de M., & Alfinito, S. (2019). Purchase intention of organic food under the influence of attributes, consumer trust and perceived value. Revista de Gestão, 26(3), 198–211. https://doi.org/10.1108/REGE-01-2018-0010

DuPuis, E. M., & Goodman, D. (2005). Should we go "home" to eat?: Toward a reflexive politics of localism. *Journal of Rural Studies, 21*(3), 359–371. https://doi.org/10.1016/J.JRURSTUD.2005.05.011

Ericksen, P. J. (2008). Conceptualizing food systems for global environmental change research. *Global Environmental Change, 18*(1), 234–245. https://doi.org/10.1016/j.gloenvcha.2007.09.002

Feliciano, R. J., Guzmán-Luna, P., Hospido, A., & Membré, J.-M. (2024). A multicriteria assessment of food safety measures for a large dairy farm in hot weather conditions. *Microbial Risk Analysis, 27–28*, 100312. https://doi.org/10.1016/j.mran.2024.100312

Funtowicz, S. O., & Ravetz, J. R. (1993). Science for the post-normal age. *Futures, 25*(7), 739–755. https://doi.org/10.1016/0016-3287(93)90022-L

Funtowicz, S. O., & Ravetz, J. R. (1994). Emergent complex systems. *Futures, 26*(6), 568–582. https://doi.org/10.1016/0016-3287(94)90029-9

Funtowicz, S., & Ravetz, J. (1990a). Post normal science: A new science for new times. *Scientific European, 266*, 20–22.

Funtowicz, S., & Ravetz, J. (1990b). *Uncertainty and quality in science for policy*. Kluwer Academic Publishers.

Gallie, W. B. (1994). Essentially contested concepts. *Inquiry: Critical Thinking Across the Disciplines, 14*(1), 3–18. https://doi.org/10.5840/inquiryctnews19941415

Giampietro, M. (2004). *Multi-scale integrated analysis of agroecosystems*. CRC Press.

Giampietro, M., Allen, T. F. H., & Mayumi, K. (2006). The epistemological predicament associated with purposive quantitative analysis. *Ecological Complexity, 3*(4), 307–327. https://doi.org/10.1016/j.ecocom.2007.02.005

Giampietro, M., & Bukkens, S. G. F. (2015). Quality assurance of knowledge claims in governance for sustainability: Transcending the duality of passion vs. reason. *International Journal of Sustainable Development, 18*(4), 282. https://doi.org/10.1504/IJSD.2015.072662

Giraldeau, L. A. (2010). Group Foraging. *Encyclopedia of Animal Behavior, Volume-Three Set*, *2*, V2–606-V2–610. https://doi.org/10.1016/B978-0-08-045337-8.00215-1

Harder, R., Giampietro, M., & Smukler, S. (2021). Towards a circular nutrient economy. A novel way to analyze the circularity of nutrient flows in food systems. *Resources, Conservation and Recycling, 172*, 105693. https://doi.org/10.1016/j.resconrec.2021.105693

Hellstrand, S. (2006). A multi-criteria analysis of sustainability effects of increasing concentrate intensity in Swedish Milk production 1989–1999. *Environment, Development and Sustainability, 8*(3), 351–373. https://doi.org/10.1007/s10668-005-6980-4

IFOAM Organics Europe. (2023). *IFOAM Organics Europe's Annual Report 2023*. https://read.organicseurope.bio/publication/ifoam-organics-europe-annual-report-2023/pdf/

Kasriel-Alexander, D. (2016). *Top 10 Global Consumer Trends for 2016*. https://twncarat.wpcomstaging.com/wp-content/uploads/2019/05/48a3b-wp_top-10-gct-2016_1.3-0116.pdf

Kato, H., Shimasaki, T., & Yayou, K. (2024). Simulations of future trends in welfare-centric egg production systems: Impacts on productivity and prices. *The Journal of Poultry Science, 61*, 2024019. https://doi.org/10.2141/jpsa.2024019

Kjærnes, U. (2012). Ethics and action: A relational perspective on consumer choice in the European politics of food. *Journal of Agricultural and Environmental Ethics, 25*(2), 145–162. https://doi.org/10.1007/S10806-011-9315-5/METRICS

Lakoff, G. (2010). Why it matters how we frame the environment. *Environmental Communication, 4*(1), 70–81. https://doi.org/10.1080/17524030903529749

Lang, T., & Barling, D. (2012). Food security and food sustainability: Reformulating the debate. *The Geographical Journal, 178*(4), 313–326. https://doi.org/10.1111/j.1475-4959.2012.00480.x

Laursen, K. B., & Noe, E. (2017). The hybrid media of economy and moral: A Luhmannian perspective on value-based-food-chains. *Journal of Rural Studies, 56*, 21–29. https://doi.org/10.1016/J.JRURSTUD.2017.09.004

Li, S., & Kallas, Z. (2021). Meta-analysis of consumers' willingness to pay for sustainable food products. *Appetite, 163*, 105239. https://doi.org/10.1016/J.APPET.2021.105239

Lusk, J. L. (2011). The market for animal welfare. *Agriculture and Human Values, 28*(4), 561–575. https://doi.org/10.1007/s10460-011-9318-x

Lusk, J. L., & Norwood, F. B. (2011). Animal welfare economics. *Applied Economic Perspectives and Policy, 33*(4), 463–483. https://doi.org/10.1093/aepp/ppr036

Manyukhina, Y. (2017). Consumer food ethics: Considerations of vulnerability, suffering, and harm. *Journal of Agricultural and Environmental Ethics, 30*(4), 595–614. https://doi.org/10.1007/S10806-017-9689-0/TABLES/1

Martinez, S., Hand, M., Da Pra, M., Pollack, S., Ralston, K., Smith, T., Vogel, S., Clark, S., Lohr, L., Low, S., & Newman, C. (2010). *Local Food Systems: Concepts, Impacts, and Issues, ERR-97*. https://ers.usda.gov/sites/default/files/_laserfiche/publications/110957/ERR-97.pdf

Mazzetto, F., & Bonera, R. (2003). MEACROS: A tool for multi-criteria evaluation of alternative cropping systems. *European Journal of Agronomy, 18*(3–4), 379–387. https://doi.org/10.1016/S1161-0301(02)00127-2

McMichael, P. (2000). The power of food. *Agriculture and Human Values, 17*(1), 21–33. https://doi.org/10.1023/A:1007684827140

Mill, J. S. (1879). *Utilitarianism*. The Floating Press. https://www.utilitarianism.com/jsmill-utilitarianism.pdf

Morgan, K. (2010). Local and green, global and fair: The ethical foodscape and the politics of care. *Environment and Planning A: Economy and Space, 42*(8), 1852–1867. https://doi.org/10.1068/a42364

Munda, G. (2004). Social multi-criteria evaluation: Methodological foundations and operational consequences. *European Journal of Operational Research, 158*(3), 662–677. https://doi.org/10.1016/S0377-2217(03)00369-2

Munda, G. (2008). *Social Multi-Criteria Evaluation for a Sustainable Economy* [Book]. Springer-Verlag Berlin Heidelberg. https://doi.org/10.1007/978-3-540-73703-2

Murdoch, J., Marsden, T., & Banks, J. (2000). Quality, nature, and embeddedness: Some theoretical considerations in the context of the food sector*. *Economic Geography, 76*(2), 107–125. https://doi.org/10.1111/j.1944-8287.2000.tb00136.x

Mustapa, M. A. C., & Kallas, Z. (2025). Meta-analysis of consumer willingness to pay for short food supply chain products. *Global Challenges, 9*(3), 2400154. https://doi.org/10.1002/GCH2.202400154

Olsen, J. V., Christensen, T., Denver, S., & Sandøe, P. (2024). Why is welfare pork so expensive? *Animal, 18*(9), 101289. https://doi.org/10.1016/j.animal.2024.101289

Paloviita, A. (2010). Consumers' sustainability perceptions of the supply chain of locally produced food. *Sustainability 2010, Vol. 2, Pages 1492–1509, 2*(6), 1492–1509. https://doi.org/10.3390/SU2061492

Porter, M. E., & Kramer, M. R. (2011). The big idea, creating shared value: How to reinvent capitalism-and unleash a wave of innovation and growth. *Harvard Business Review.*. https://www.communitylivingbc.ca/wp-content/uploads/2018/05/Creating-Shared-Value.pdf

Reinert, E. S. (2007). *How rich countries got rich—and why poor countries stay poor*. Constable.

Röling, N., & Wagemakers, A. (1998). *Facilitating sustainable agriculture: Participatory learning and adaptive management in times of environmental uncertainty*. Cambridge University Press.

Saltelli, A., Benini, L., Funtowicz, S., Giampietro, M., Kaiser, M., Reinert, E., & van der Sluijs, J. P. (2020). The technique is never neutral. How methodological choices condition the generation of narratives for sustainability. *Environmental Science & Policy, 106*, 87–98. https://doi.org/10.1016/j.envsci.2020.01.008

Schrobback, P., Zhang, A., Loechel, B., Ricketts, K., & Ingham, A. (2023). Food Credence Attributes: A Conceptual Framework of Supply Chain

Stakeholders, Their Motives, and Mechanisms to Address Information Asymmetry. *Foods 2023, Vol. 12, Page 538, 12*(3), 538. https://doi.org/10.3390/FOODS12030538

Scuderi, A., & Sturiale, L. (2016). Multi-criteria evaluation model to face phytosanitary emergencies: The case of citrus fruits farming in Italy. *Agricultural Economics (Zemědělská Ekonomika), 62*(5), 205–214. https://doi.org/10.17221/114/2015-AGRICECON

Sgroi, F., Sciortino, C., Baviera-Puig, A., & Modica, F. (2024). Analyzing consumer trends in functional foods: A cluster analysis approach. *Journal of Agriculture and Food Research, 15*, 101041. https://doi.org/10.1016/J.JAFR.2024.101041

Sjöström, K., Sternberg-Lewerin, S., Blanco-Penedo, I., Duval, J. E., Krieger, M., Emanuelson, U., & Fall, N. (2019). Effects of a participatory approach, with systematic impact matrix analysis in herd health planning in organic dairy cattle herds. *Animal, 13*(2), 358–366. https://doi.org/10.1017/S1751731118002008

Sobal, J., Kettel Khan, L., & Bisogni, C. (1998). A conceptual model of the food and nutrition system. *Social Science & Medicine, 47*(7), 853–863. https://doi.org/10.1016/S0277-9536(98)00104-X

Sonnino, R., & Marsden, T. (2006). Beyond the divide: Rethinking relationships between alternative and conventional food networks in Europe. *Journal of Economic Geography, 6*(2), 181–199. https://doi.org/10.1093/jeg/lbi006

Springmann, M. (2024). A multicriteria analysis of meat and milk alternatives from nutritional, health, environmental, and cost perspectives. *Proceedings of the National Academy of Sciences, 121*(50). https://doi.org/10.1073/pnas.2319010121

Stephens, D. W., & Krebs, J. R. (1986). *Foraging Theory*. Princeton University Press. doi:https://doi.org/10.2307/j.ctvs32s6b.

Stirling, A. (2003). Risk, uncertainty and precaution: Some instrumental implications from the social sciences. In F. Berkhout, M. Leach, & I. Scoones (Eds.), *Negotiating environmental change—new perspectives from social science*. Edward Elgar Publishing. https://doi.org/10.4337/9781843765653.00008

Stolz, H., Stolze, M., Hamm, U., Janssen, M., & Ruto, E. (2011). Consumer attitudes towards organic versus conventional food with specific quality attributes. *NJAS: Wageningen Journal of Life Sciences, 58*(3–4), 67–72. https://doi.org/10.1016/j.njas.2010.10.002

Tandon, A., Dhir, A., Kaur, P., Kushwah, S., & Salo, J. (2020). Behavioral reasoning perspectives on organic food purchase. *Appetite, 154*, 104786. https://doi.org/10.1016/j.appet.2020.104786

Tansey, G., & Rajotte, T. (Eds.). (2008). *The future control of food: A guide to international negotiations and rules on intellectual property*. Biodiversity and Food Security. https://scispace.com/pdf/the-future-control-of-food-37wgt0aw06.pdf

Tilman, D., & Clark, M. (2014). Global diets link environmental sustainability and human health. *Nature, 515*(7528), 518–522. https://doi.org/10.1038/nature13959

United States Department of Agriculture (USDA), National Agricultural Statistics Service (NASS). (2025). *Milk Production Survey: Milk Production July 2025* (data released August 21, 2025). https://downloads.usda.library.cornell.edu/usda-esmis/files/h989r321c/kw52m9004/np1958813/mkpr0825.pdf. See also https://usda.library.cornell.edu/concern/publications/h989r321c?locale=en (Accessed September 18th, 2025).

Vivero-Pol, J. L. (2017). Food as Commons or Commodity? Exploring the Links between Normative Valuations and Agency in Food Transition. *Sustainability 2017, Vol. 9, Page 442*, *9*(3), 442. https://doi.org/10.3390/SU9030442

Vorley, B. (2003). *Food, Inc.: Corporate concentration from farm to consumer*. https://www.ukfg.org.uk/files/UKFG_FoodInc_2003.pdf

Wang, J. M., Liu, Q., Hou, Y., Qin, W., Bai, Z. H., Zhang, F. S., & Oenema, O. (2022). Impacts of international food and feed trade on nitrogen balances and nitrogen use efficiencies of food systems. *Science of the Total Environment, 838*, 156151. https://doi.org/10.1016/j.scitotenv.2022.156151

Wu, W., Zhang, A., van Klinken, R. D., Schrobback, P., & Muller, J. M. (2021). Consumer Trust in Food and the food system: A critical review. *Food, 10*(10), 2490. https://doi.org/10.3390/foods10102490

Yussefi-Menzler, M. (2010). In H. Willer & N. Sorensen (Eds.), *The world of organic agriculture*. Routledge. https://doi.org/10.4324/9781849775991

Ethics and Communication

Opportunities and Problems with Cultured Meat

Adriano Fabris

1 Good Eating, Bad Eating

The approach we usually take to what is a source of nourishment for humans is, more often than not, a two-pronged approach. In a nutshell, it leads to the following alternative: either we focus on our personal taste, on what the *subject* needs or likes, or we end up fetishising the *object,* the source of food, and eventually making it, in some respects, untouchable. The former is the *gourmand*'s stance, the latter is the stance of those who, for some specific reasons, do not want to feed on some foods and often ask others to abstain themselves.

It is an antithetical approach, quite frequently taken to the extreme. It can be seen in some *slow food* enthusiasts' positions or in some vegan attitudes. In this regard, we need to broaden our horizons. The way we can do that is by starting all over again, even in our decisions around

A. Fabris (✉)
Department of Civilisation and Forms of Knowledge, University of Pisa, Pisa, Italy
e-mail: adriano.fabris@unipi.it

F. Bruno et al. (eds.), *Healthcare and Food,*
https://doi.org/10.1007/978-981-95-5899-5_4

food, not from the subject or object of the food relationship, but from the relationship itself: from the fact, in other words, that any being is one side of a relationship, a being connected with other beings. And this applies not just to the eater but to what can provide nourishment as well. At an ecological level, the consequences of such a position are clear, and I will refer to them anyway in what I am going to say later on.

In other words, the key issue we need to address is not just the alternative between assimilating otherness and prohibiting, in some or all cases, such assimilation, that is, the alternative between the self-affirmation of a subject—i.e. usually the human subject—and the protection of other beings at all costs. This is about building a good, well-balanced relationship between all the parties involved. More precisely, this is about understanding what "good", "well-balanced" mean in this case, and how to accomplish this in our daily habits: even, and above all, in the behaviours that have to do with our survival. But to do this, I insist, we need to broaden our horizons.

The way I will try to do this will revolve around cultured meat as a case study. I will try to shed light on the connections such topic leads into. I will show that, to properly understand it, not only do we have to broaden our horizons, we also need to expand the semantics of the words we use when we talk about it. Lastly, I will show how such technological innovation can help us shed light on some basic ethical principles, which can be shared by anyone and allow us to really understand what eating "well" means.

2 A Relational Approach to Food

The topic that frames my argument and that I have addressed in some of my recent books (see, above all, Fabris, 2024) is the transition from a one-sided approach to a relational approach to food. A food is good, ethically good, not because some subject likes it or because its source is protected and respected, but because it is part of a good relationship. The relationship is good, ethically good, insofar as it is fruitful, productive, open to other relationships. A relationship is bad, ethically bad, insofar as it destroys the possibility to maintain, develop, implement such relationships.

If we apply such a definition to eating (and, albeit differently, to drinking), we find that, as we feed ourselves, a relationship is wiped off. Those who eat assimilate and, therefore, they destroy: they destroy the other one, they destroy the possibility of a relationship with that other one, which is the source of food. But another question comes to the fore here, which our philosophical inquiry sheds light on. To ethically address this question, we need to consider the entirety of relationships. One cannot just consider a relationship with something specific or analyse a specific form of relationship (as both the *gourmand* and the vegan, that we have taken as the two extremes of the food relationship, actually do). Neither can one fixate on a single relationship. Every relationship, as such, is tied up with other relationships: it is a relationship just because it is part of a context of other relationships and interacts with them. That's why we need to broaden our horizons and identify all the implications, or at least those we can address, of the relationships in which we are more closely involved. Such approach allows us to ethically regulate food relationships too. Here, "ethically" is tied up—I repeat—with the principle whereby a relationship is good insofar as it promotes relationships and situates a behaviour within the overall context of the relationships it is involved in.

However, the situation is further complicated in the high-tech scenario we are living in. Technology expands our relational skills. At the same time, though, it also steers them and may turn them into a one-sided something (Elliott, 2018). I mean, technology conforms to one single form of relationship, the procedure-based one, and only promotes some meanings and some forms of relationship. They include forms associated with the production of something, the achievement of profitable goals. This is about standardising a behaviour based on effectiveness and efficiency. This applies to our food relationships as well. So, we need to delve deeper, at least in some respects, into what changes in our food relationship in the high-tech scenario we live in.

To do this, as I mentioned, I will deal with the specific case of cultured meat. I will try to show the multiple relational intersections that are inherent in such technological innovation for the agricultural industry, where large-scale production, safety certification, and reduction of marketing costs are still largely underdeveloped. I will start by looking into the resemanticisation and expansion of our language, so as to be able to speak of "meat" even in this connection: in relation to what such product is and looks like.[1]

3 Extending the Semantics

Technological advances extend the meanings of the words we use. In that way, they introduce ambiguities, which need to be handled. This happens, for example, when we speak, now more than ever, of "artificial intelligence". This also happens when we speak of "cultured meat". For our purposes, continuing such parallel comparison may be helpful.

Is artificial intelligence *intelligence*, or is it not? Is cultured meat *meat*, or is it not? In both cases, we could answer "yes" and "no". We can, insofar as we specify in what way they are and in what way they are not. Most importantly, we can, insofar as we understand the mechanism that in both cases underlies such extension of meaning I mentioned above.

Artificial intelligence is understood to be "intelligence" insofar as software can be qualified as such, in other words, software can be understood as being "intelligent", it performs in ways that might be confused with some human behaviours. This is how the Turing Test works (Turing, 1950). Eventually, with the developments of *machine learning*, *deep learning* and generative artificial intelligence, some devices have not only outperformed our brain (in terms of speed, data management, and data processing capacity), they have further developed such abilities by adding more skills to their original performance and claiming therefore to be interchangeable with us.

There is still a basic difference, though. Machines may be programmed, they can learn, they can change their "behaviours", they can act with some autonomy, but they cannot programme themselves.

[1] For an insight into philosophical issues around such topic, see, in Italian: (Benanti, 2017; Bondi 2022; Lo Sapio 2024). The books in English are the most useful, even if mainly introductory in character: see for example (Aldes Wurgaft 2019; Shapiro 2024).

In other words, unlike humans, they cannot change the criteria for their actions and reflect on the principles that guide and steer them. They have no self-reference, either theoretically or ethically (Andler, 2023).

There lies the similarity, and there lies the difference between artificial intelligence and human intelligence. Put it this way, even artificial entities can be qualified as "intelligent" but up to a point. The limits and features of human and artificial entities are the result of their differences. There's a fairly similar behaviour, at least in terms of results-based performance, a fairly different one. Actually, the relationships that machines promote are relationships based on effectiveness and efficiency: therefore, based on usefulness. Humans instead promote many different types of relationships, even if they may be useless or otherwise useful. Humans are in the position to promote them because they are always involved in them. In other words, programmes only work procedurally. Humans have very cogent processes, instead.

Something similar happens with the so-called "cultured meat" or "lab-grown meat". Is it really meat? Yes, because it is sourced, through specific culturing processes, from animal stem cells. So, it really is meat. However, it is not a meat that has grown through, so to speak, a "natural" process, because it has been synthesised, "lab-grown" through such processes.

The result is a product that can still be interchanged with "natural" meat. It is edible meat. It is consumed as food. Of course: there may be specific problems that, if occurring in the "culturing" process, can alter the edibleness of the product or make it harmful to health. But these are problems that can be solved by future technological advances. From this perspective, then, we can say we have to do with meat: even if—in the way it is produced, not the purpose it serves—it is a different meat, it is "another" meat.

After all, as much with artificial intelligence as with cultured meat, we have no other words to speak of new entities. If we look at the results, we must call the two products "intelligence" and "meat", respectively. We will still try to soften the meaning of the noun with a qualifying adjective. In the former case, we will speak of "artificial" intelligence, in the latter case we will speak of "cultured" or "lab-grown" meat. But the power of the noun will still affect our understanding of the phenomenon, pushing us to identify human intelligence with the intelligence attributed to some software and animal meat with lab-grown meat.

There is an illusion in all this, but there are alarm bells ringing too. The illusion is that we too have managed to create something similar, if not downright identical, to what used to be a product of nature. Once again, we seem to arrogate to ourselves the right to be creator gods (Wiener, 1966). The risk is that we might realise that what we have created is not, after all, so similar to what is natural. And it is when we perceive such difference that we feel ill at ease with, if not actually afraid of, such entities.

4 The Pros and Cons of Cultured Meat

This is precisely what happened with cultured meat. And actually, at least in Italy, the production and sale of cultured meat have been banned. There are several reasons for that. As to the measure taken by the Italian Parliament, it is mainly due to the idea that the production of artificial, "fake" foods (such as "parmesan" instead of Parmigiano) would undermine the goodness, specificity, and naturalness of Italian products. Farmers, butchers, wholesale and retail sellers would be the first to be damaged by such a situation. It would jeopardise food sovereignty, controlled designations of foods, it would even jeopardise jobs: at least as far as some traditional uses are concerned.

In fact, the arguments against cultured meat are even more, many more. They are mainly psychological arguments. Sometimes, they are ethical arguments. They range from revulsion at something that lies beyond our usual confines to the risk that such practice may be extended beyond the production of animal meat. Actually, with a bit of a stretch, human cells could be synthesised and eaten too, thus making cannibalism possible (and legal too, even more so because human meat could be sourced in a nonviolent way). I could even synthetise my own cells, thus making autophagia possible (and legal). But one could perhaps get used to all this, as it happened in other circumstances before, or it could be carefully regulated, as it happened with other technological innovations.

At a psychological level, the real issue is our resistance to what can replace a naturally organic entity with something that is artificially so. Here, we are not dealing with—as in the case of artificial intelligence—an entity that, in many respects, functions in the same way as the one it intends to imitate—i.e. human intelligence—even ontologically different from it. Here, we are dealing with something artificial that, just because of what it is, just because of its features, can cater to the same needs as those that are met by what is natural. On cultured meat, we feed in the same way, and through it we experience the same form of food relationship we experience when we eat animal meat, for instance. In other words, here the identification between the two entities and the successful replacement of the organic with the synthetic are accomplished, confirmed, certified in the very assimilation that we submit cultured meat to. We make something artificial our own—in other words, we sort of "naturalise" something artificial.

Throughout their history, instead, humans have usually followed a different path. To feed themselves they grew organic. Namely, by submitting it to specific practices, they transformed what naturally grew in the wild into something artificially produced. From hunters and gatherers to farmers. But, in this case, the organic, albeit manipulated, remained such in the end. It was transformed, implemented, hybridised, but it did not lose its underlying character, its nature. It was intensively reproduced and improved in terms of crop yields, it was the outcome of a technical process but it was always called the same, without any problems: grains, fruits, vegetables.

Now, the process is different. Parts of sentient beings are reproduced into non-sentient parts to serve our nutritional purposes, which is good and bad, at the same time. It is good because, if we go this way, we don't have to kill to feed ourselves and maybe have other sentient beings suffer while they are being raised. It is bad, because such beings are treated as elements to be manipulated anyway. From the outset, they are conceived as parts, pieces, components, not in the complexity and entirety of their being as organisms. So, the respect for living beings, viewed just as such, dies down: as much as the respect of the human being for the organic vegetable world has been dying down for quite a while now, in many of his behaviours.

However, despite all this, there are quite a few moral arguments in support of cultured meat. We know them, but I'll briefly repeat them. As I said, it could be an answer to intensive breeding. It could provide human with a carnivore diet while steering clear of vegetarian and vegan arguments. It could reduce the problem of world hunger.

Of course: the production of cultured meat is still too complex and too expensive for the time being. But technological innovations will soon cause the price to fall and the food to be within everyone's means. As long as no monopoly position is established by one or more producers, as it often happened in the past, so that the profits are reaped by the happy few.

5 Additional Benefits of Cultured Meat

The debate on the pros and cons of cultured meat, even and above all from a moral standpoint, is in fact even wider and fiercer. But here I will not linger on such debate. In conclusion, I want to propose, instead, an ulterior motive, or better a number of motives, that can lead us, despite the doubts I had before, to justify the consumption of cultured meat in an ethical, shared way. I mean to do this by taking a relational approach to the matter: the approach I briefly mentioned at the beginning to get out of the alternative between subjectification and objectification of food.

How can the consumption of cultured meat be relationally justified? How can we approach a good use of cultured meat, in such a way? Firstly, it can be done by not fetishising the object and at the same time by not condemning a given product as a matter of principle. On the contrary, we must focus on the relationship we have with it, weigh how fruitful it can be in promoting other relationships, and thus place such relationship, by broadening our horizons, within an overall relational context: not just a nutritional one, but a downright ecological one.

There is no doubt that, from such a perspective, cultured meat can have its advantages. If human beings need to assimilate other living beings—all sorts of living beings: plants and animals—to survive and if to such end they have to thwart the free development of the living beings they feed on—and this applies not only to animals in intensive farms or even those that are free to roam or live in the wild, which are still bound to be killed for food, it applies as much to vegetables, which are life forms themselves anyway—the only way not to destroy other beings and not give up human survival is synthetic food, as an all-encompassing term. And, among all forms of synthetic foods, cultured meat could perhaps meet our needs better than most. I am speaking of nutritional needs, taste preferences, ethical and ecological requirements.

First and foremost, such option could fulfil the nutritional requirements of human beings. There would be no problem reproducing beef proteins for assimilation. At least on the surface, the nutritional intake would be the same as that of meat sourced from raised or hunted animals. Actually, from this point of view, there could be improvements in the process of growing synthetic meat by adding elements that could further benefit our health.

Cultured meat can then meet the taste preferences of humans. The flavour, the pleasure of food should not be restrained, provided it does not clash with other beliefs that humans uphold themselves. It should certainly not be glorified, it cannot be the only reason to eat at the expense of everything else—as it may happen, for instance, in *slow food* communities (Petrini & Padovani, 2006)—but it cannot be denied either, since human beings not only have to live, they can live both pleasantly (and this is better than living unpleasantly) and ethically (i.e. in a non-destructive relationship with other beings). At any rate, a lab-grown burger can certainly be tastier than a pill.

Moreover, such kind of nutrition can meet the ethical requirements that we can specifically embrace. Not only can it oppose to the violence inherent in the assimilation of the beings we feed on, it can allow us to try out other ways of feeding ourselves, by reproducing old practices and defining new ones. Most importantly, though, based on the relational principle—the one that accounts for the ethics of our behaviours—the consumption of cultured meat would not break our relationships with other beings: those bound to be eaten. It would not involve the destruction of other living beings, either animals or plants. Actually, by eating that way, it would make us experience additional opportunities to build relationships.

Finally, the consumption of cultured meat can or could meet our ecological requirements. This should be even better explained in practical terms. It should mainly be specified in terms of production process and effects. However, we might expect such effects to be less remarkable and impactful than those of intensive breeding, in terms of pollution as well as in terms of destroying other living beings. However, this is a question that needs to be carefully checked and promoted.

6 Conclusions: Expanding the Horizons

In conclusion, even in this case, namely the consumption of cultured meat, the horizon-expanding method allows us not to focus entirely on one single relationship with a given food, but makes us take into account the other relationships we have with human beings (such as: reducing world hunger), with other living beings (e.g. they would not be subjected to intensive farming or hunting practices), with ourselves (we could feed ourselves without harming any other being or the entire ecosystem) as well. Framed this way, the relationship turns out to be a good one, because it will not break but will promote other relationships. In so doing, even the act of eating can lose its violent connotation, destructive of other living beings and—by assimilation of an entity that turns out to be as much living as non-living, organic but not natural—it can promote a nutrition experience for us human beings through which we can find ourselves in an even deeper symbiotic relationship with the other beings.

References

Aldes Wurgaft, B. (2019). *Meat planet. Artificial flesh and the future of food.* University of California Press.

Andler, D. (2023). *Intelligence artificielle, intelligence humaine: le double énigme.* Gallimard.

Benanti, P. (2017). *L'hamburger di Frankenstein. La rivoluzione della carne sintetica*. EDB.

Bondi, D. (2022). Coltivare la carne. Considerazioni etico-ontologiche sulla cultured meat. *Teoria*, 2022/1, issue devoted to *Food and Philosophy/Cibo e filosofia*.

Elliott, A. (2018). *The culture of AI: Everyday life and digital revolution*. Routledge.

Fabris, A. (2024). *Ethics of eating and drinking*. Springer.

Lo Sapio, L. (2024). *Carne coltivata. Etica dell'agricoltura cellulare*. Carocci.

Petrini, C., & Padovani, G. (2006). *Slow food revolution. A new culture for eating and living*. Rizzoli.

Shapiro, P. (2024). *Clean meat: How growing meat without animals will revolutionize dinner and the world*. Gallery Books.

Turing, A. (1950). Computing machinery and intelligence. *Mind, 59*(236), 433–460.

Wiener, N. (1966). *God & Golem Inc: A comment on certain points where cybernetics impinges on religion*. The MIT Press.

Behavioral Paternalism and Food Ethics: Political Justifications beyond Nudges and Public Reason

Giacomo Brioni, Jacopo Marchetti, and Antonio Masala

1 Introduction

In recent years, nudge-based approaches have become a central topic in ethics and public policy, particularly in areas related to health and personal well-being. Promoted as a means of influencing individual behavior without restricting freedom of choice, Behavioral Paternalism (BP) relies on the use of nudges to steer individuals toward decisions that are presumed to align with their best interests. Unlike other branches of behavioral economics that remain neutral or skeptical about policy intervention, BP explicitly advocates for the application of behavioral

G. Brioni (✉) · J. Marchetti · A. Masala
Department of Civilisation and Forms of Knowledge, University of Pisa, Pisa, Italy
e-mail: giacomo.brioni@phd.unipi.it

J. Marchetti
e-mail: jacopo.marchetti@cfs.unipi.it

A. Masala
e-mail: antonio.masala@unipi.it

F. Bruno et al. (eds.), *Healthcare and Food*,
https://doi.org/10.1007/978-981-95-5899-5_5

insights in decision-making contexts, especially where individuals are prone to cognitive biases or bounded rationality. The core aim is to help people make choices that reflect their genuine preferences, without removing any options from consideration (Congiu & Moscati, 2022). This approach encompasses a wide range of policy tools. Notable examples include cooling-off periods designed to curb impulsive purchases, graphic health warnings on cigarette packaging, and labels such as Protected Designation of Origin (PDO) that help consumers distinguish high-quality food products from generic or lower-grade alternatives. In particular, the debate on nudging has increasingly entered the field of food ethics. A central question that arises is whether it is ethically and politically justifiable to employ behavioral tools to influence individuals' dietary choices—encouraging them to adopt healthier and more environmentally sustainable habits (Barnhill & Civita, 2020). As eating habits are closely tied to autonomous choices, cultural practices, and notions of the good life, this domain poses especially challenging questions about autonomy, welfare, and the legitimate scope of public intervention.

These debates highlight the growing relevance of food ethics, an emerging interdisciplinary field that explores the moral, social, and political dimensions of food production, distribution, and consumption. As food policy becomes an increasingly contested arena, food ethics provides a critical framework for navigating the complex intersection of health, equity, and individual autonomy. While nudging is often presented as a non-coercive form of political guidance, it raises important concerns: Does it truly respect individual autonomy, particularly the autonomy to choose what to eat—including the choice to eat unhealthily? Moreover, how can we, from a political perspective, balance individual freedom with public health objectives? These tensions lie at the heart of contemporary discussions on ethical food policy. However, the political implications of these issues remain less explored than their ethical and moral dimensions.

This chapter seeks to broaden the scope of the debate by critically examining the claims made by advocates of behavioral paternalism, particularly in connection with the objections raised by scholars such as Robert Sugden, Mario J. Rizzo, and Glenn Whitman (Section 2). According to them, BP rests on a problematic reading of behavioral economics. In their view, it often misrepresents empirical findings and ultimately smuggles back into policy discourse the normative assumptions of the standard model of the rational actor. Nudging, in this sense, becomes a means of covertly reimposing idealized rationality onto real agents, rather than accommodating their actual cognitive and motivational attitudes. From a political and moral theory standpoint, BP tends to subordinate individuals' real preferences—and the diverse conceptions of the good life those preferences reflect—to the values or goals of policymakers. Despite its libertarian label, we state that BP may ultimately erode the space for autonomous decision-making by replacing individual ends with externally defined ones, however benevolent the intention.

The ethical and political tensions associated with BP are especially pronounced in food policy, where dietary decisions are intertwined with a complex web of values including pleasure, tradition, culture, autonomy, and identity (Section 3). This complexity makes food-related interventions particularly susceptible to criticisms of paternalism, even when such policies are framed as non-coercive. Barnhill and Bonotti (2022) provide an important alternative perspective, arguing that food policies need not be paternalistic if they are justified through public reason and designed to promote collective, rather than individual, ends. As we shall see, their model emphasizes legitimacy based on procedural norms that ensure reasons are accessible to citizens with diverse moral and political views, supported by decentralized deliberative mechanisms such as citizens' deliberative polls. However, this approach faces significant challenges: it still assumes institutions can interpret or respect individuals' ends, and struggles to fully address the layered and plural motivations underlying food choices. Consequently, procedural consensus may be unattainable.

We will then shift the focus to the political implications of the debate on BP and food ethics (Section 4). This section adopts a publicly oriented perspective on dietary behavior, focusing on the societal impact of unhealthy eating. Rather than framing the issue in moral or paternalistic terms, it presents healthy eating policies as responses to coordination and collective action problems. A paradigmatic example is the strain placed on publicly funded healthcare systems by widespread unhealthy consumption, which leads to higher rates of preventable illness, increased demand for care, and rising public costs, raising concerns about resource allocation and tax burden distribution.

2 Why Does Nudging Miss the Mark on Autonomy? Drawing from Sugden and Rizzo

While various forms of paternalism existed prior to the emergence of nudges, the latter represent the most appealing and innovative development in paternalistic approaches, especially following the landmark publication by Thaler and Sunstein (2003). According to one line of thought, paternalistic intervention is justifiable insofar as individuals lack genuine voluntariness in their actions. An alternative perspective, however, maintains that even fully voluntary behaviors may warrant paternalistic regulation, particularly when such behaviors stem from misinformation, cognitive biases, or irrational judgment (Aird, 2023; Conly, 2013; Trout, 2005; Turner, 2024). Although libertarian paternalism has gained considerable traction in the field of behavioral normative policy-making, several influential scholars have recently questioned whether its findings are legitimated to support broad policy applications, particularly when behavioral insights are used to justify nudge-based interventions (Entwistle, 2021; Gigerenzer, 2015; Grüne-Yanoff, 2012; Grüne-Yanoff & Hertwig, 2016; Hausman & Welch, 2010; Kuyer & Gordijn, 2023; Oliver, 2023; Viale, 2022). In addition, new forms of paternalism have emerged, most notably BP. This approach creates the impression that behaviors traditionally deemed biased because they divert from the normative standards of rational choice theory should be corrected through nudges designed by behavioral economists and policy-makers (Rizzo, 2016). The works of Rizzo and Whitman (2019) and Sugden (2018) stand out as the most comprehensive critiques of behavioral paternalism, highlighting its epistemic and practical shortcomings. The authors present a robust critique of BP from multiple perspectives.

The first line of criticism concerns the concept of rationality, a concept that economists have struggled with for a long time. BP rejects the neoclassical model of individuals as utility-maximizing agents, yet it continues to evaluate human behavior against the very same normative standard of rationality embedded in that model. As a result, individuals are deemed 'not fully rational' when they deviate from it. In this sense, BP absorbs the foundational critique of behavioral economics, which takes aim at the 'standard model' of rational choice theory, also known as "substantive rationality", as opposed to "procedural rationality" (Simon, 1976). Since the complete optimization of means to achieve given ends would require abilities more akin to those of a deity than a human being—saying it in Herbert A. Simon's terms, it would demand "olympian rationality"—human behavior ought to be understood through the lens of bounded rationality. This concept has inspired a wide range of subsequent research, which has developed in two main directions. On the one hand, bounded rationality has been interpreted as an erosion of the assumptions of full rationality (Kahneman, 2003; Tversky & Kahneman, 1974). On the other, it has been understood as an alternative model of decision-making, not necessarily inferior, but structurally different from optimization (Gigerenzer, 2004; Gigerenzer & Gaissmaier, 2011). Behavioral paternalism appears to overlook the cognitive implications of the latter interpretation, clinging instead to a standard of rationality that bounded rationality was meant to replace.

Rizzo and Whitman welcome the insights offered by behavioral economics and the social sciences, particularly the effort to take human behavior seriously by shifting "attention to the study of Humans rather than Econs" (Thaler, 2016: 1597). However, they also argue that "despite having rejected rationality as a model of how people do behave, the behavioral paternalists still accept rationality as a model of how people *ought* to behave" (Rizzo & Whitman, 2019: 16). In doing so, BP has been too quick to move from descriptive analyses to normative conclusions in support of paternalistic policies, falling into the error of "conflating their models with reality—and, when reality fails to conform to the model, judging it deficient" (Rizzo & Whitman, 2019: 180). Put simply, behavioral paternalism implicitly assumes from the outset a strong normative stance—that the 'right' way to make decisions requires cognitive and behavioral capacities that actual humans simply lack: the ability to hold complete and consistent preferences, to reason in a logically coherent and truth-tracking manner (i.e., to hold beliefs that accurately reflect the world as it is), and to reliably adapt their beliefs in response to new evidence. By this, Rizzo and Whitman mean that BP seeks "policies on the basis of people's own values and preferences". Instead, it applies "an external set of values" by taking the "neoclassical definition of rationality" (Rizzo & Whitman, 2019: 17) as a normative standard of 'good' decision-making (Dold, 2023; Dold et al., 2024).

This leads to a key point in the second line of criticism advanced by Rizzo and Whitman: behavioral paternalism tends to subordinate individuals' actual preferences to the values or objectives of policy-makers. When Rizzo and Whitman discuss the practical challenges of implementing BP, they highlight several concerns, chief among them the tendency of paternalistic policies to reflect a mixture of the policy-makers' own preferences, socially sanctioned norms, or special-interest influences—"none of which are synonymous with the real preferences of the individuals targeted by paternalistic laws" (Rizzo & Whitman, 2019: 20). In essence, BP seeks to bridge the gap between the idealized rational agent and the real, flesh-and-blood decision-maker. However, it does so in a misguided manner, as in "the rush to characterize certain 'anomalies of choice' as violations of rationality, behavioral paternalists have been insufficiently subjectivist" (Rizzo & Whitman, 2019: 317). For that reason, they tend to privilege a top-down approach that reflects the perspective of the paternalistic policy-maker, often at the expense of the individual's bottom-up, context-dependent knowledge (Boettke, 2000; Storr & John, 2020). This means that BP implicitly assumes that paternalistic policy-makers are in a position to determine what is best for individuals, thereby downplaying the importance of personal knowledge (Hayek, 1937; Polanyi, 2015; see Zappia, 1996) and agency.

The argument about the internal inconsistency of BP is also a pivotal point of Robert Sugden's analysis. Sugden positions himself in the line of inquiry opened by James M. Buchanan's critique of Utilitarian welfare economics. Buchanan (1949) criticized the welfare economics of his time for its reliance on a "benevolent despot" model of the policy-maker. The latter was conceived of as an exogenous equilibrating force, using the levers of economic policy to score the maximum aggregate utility, with the political economist playing the role of the 'prince's advisor.' On the opposite side, Buchanan thought that citizens, not policy-makers, should be the primary addressees of policy proposals (Sugden, 2018: 51). Institutions should be designed to let people pursue their own objectives without damaging others (Sugden, 2018: 19–24). To Sugden, BP marks a covert return to the Utilitarian perspective. The way Thaler and Sunstein employ the behavioral refutation of the *homo oeconomicus* model introduces an implicit cleavage between the weak-mindedness of ordinary people, subject to the perils of cognitive biases, and the supposed clarity of well-intentioned "choice architects" (Thaler & Sunstein, 2008). According to Thaler and Sunstein, the latter would operate to help people choose what they would choose if they always acted in a collected fashion. Sugden argues that this is an unwarranted conclusion: how can we determine that people are willing to be nudged, or that our image of what is a 'rational' end to pursue accurately reflects their true preferences? (Sugden, 2018: 47–50).

To Sugden, the main error of BP lies in its ontology of the choosing individual. This ontology consists of two layers. The first one is represented by those features of human behavior that are influenced by the choice context: cognitive biases interact with this superficial layer, resulting in impulsive decisions. On a deeper level lies a core of rational preferences that are the sources of long-term planning and self-control efforts—the "inner rational agent" (Sugden, 2018: ch. 4). BP advocates act as if this second layer were accessible to the policy-maker, whose task is to help individuals stick to their 'true' preferences. Sugden replies that the contributions of behavioral economics effectively deny this possibility, since they refute the very notion of "integrated preferences" (Sugden, 2018: 58). If human behavior is everywhere "context-dependent" (Sugden, 2018: 58), the individual must be conceived as a unitarian entity, with every choice bearing the same token of responsibility (Sugden, 2018: 100–106). BP, therefore, superimposes on the individual a set of ends that only reflects the policy-maker's *desiderata*.

While attempting to bridge the gap between idealized models and real-world behavior is a valuable endeavor, it remains insufficient on its own. This approach risks falling into what Rizzo and Whitman call the *nirvana fallacy* (Rizzo & Whitman, 2019: 310), namely the assumption that any deviation from an ideal standard is, in itself, a sufficient justification for paternalistic intervention. This opens the door to the third and final line of criticism, i.e., the so-called slippery-slope tendency. To Rizzo and Whitman, seemingly benign forms of paternalism can act as a gateway to more intrusive and liberty-constraining regulatory frameworks. This line of reasoning echoes Hayek's argument in *The Road to Serfdom* (Hayek, 2008), where he warns that even seemingly moderate forms of economic and social intervention, when left unchecked, can set democratic societies on a gradual path toward centralized control and totalitarian planning. According to Hayek, the danger lies not in the intentions behind interventionist policies, but in the structural logic they follow: each new intervention tends to generate unforeseen consequences that then require further state control, creating a cumulative dynamic that progressively erodes individual freedom. Similarly, although the discussion of BP starts with an emphasis on individuals' 'true' preferences, the difficulties in conceptualizing and measuring these preferences often lead to a shift from the agent's perspective to that of the paternalist policy-maker, who ends up unwittingly imposing their own values. This leads to the paradox that if withholding information is deemed to be in the best interest of individuals, then lying might also be justified—if it effectively leads them toward what policy-makers believe are their best interests. However, such an approach would be fundamentally incompatible with the core principles of liberal democracy.

To conclude, the criticisms of BP summarized above amount to a refutation of *akrasia* (e.g., Sugden, 2018: 79–81) as an adequate descriptor of human choice patterns—a contention which is especially wrong when advanced in the context of contemporary behavioral economics. Both Sugden (2018) and Rizzo and Whitman (2019) warn that the concern of BP advocates for helping people realize their 'best interests' may all too easily turn into an argument for pursuing the policy-maker's conception of what those interests are. The fact that preferences are content-indeterminate and context-dependent should function as a constraint on policy-making. However, BP mistakes these features for reasons in favor of political interventionism.

3 Paternalism or Public Reason? A Comment on Barnhill and Bonotti

Few areas of human life are more sensitive to the problem of paternalism than eating habits. Food choices are strictly related to the long-term health of the individual, but they are also the prime example many people would think of when the theme of irrationality is brought up. On the surface, we all know that a balanced diet is beneficial, but when it comes to everyday decisions we often give in to temptation and choose taste over health. Although weakness of will certainly plays a role in this scenario, it makes only for a partial explanation. The truth is that the social environment in which we make our choices is often organized—willingly or not—in order to divert our self-control. Food industries, for example, are known to spend a lot of resources for the advertisement of processed products, which therefore catch more easily the attention of customers (Barnhill & Bonotti, 2022: 11). This is where the paternalist argument comes into play: people should be steered toward making healthier eating choices through properly designed policies. It is not by chance that Thaler and Sunstein begin their book *Nudge* (2008) with a mental experiment that concerns food. Thaler and Sunstein ask us to put ourselves in the shoes of a school cafeteria manager, who is tasked with arranging the options on the counter from which the kids will choose at lunch time. There are a few principles on which she can base her decision, like maximizing the cafeteria profits or trying to promote the best options for the children's health. Thaler and Sunstein put the emphasis on the fact that the manager plays the role of the "choice architect", and that no choice environment can ever be neutral. Therefore, policy-making should be conducted to further the well-being of the actors. However, there is an obvious problem with this position: Is the policy-maker entitled to decide what is best for everybody else? In a liberal democratic framework, great value is placed on individual autonomy, and paternalism inherently contradicts this feature, as it overrides the individuals' ability to form their own conception of the good. It must be stressed that the clash between liberty and autonomy doesn't concern only libertarian paternalism: everyone who seeks to legitimize paternalistic policies in a democratic setting is bound to confront this issue.

In recent times, the most exhaustive attempt to frame the debate on food policies in terms of political philosophy and to tackle the problem of how to justify supposedly paternalist reforms has been made by Anne Barnhill and Matteo Bonotti in their book *Healthy Eating Policy and Political Philosophy: A Public Reason Approach* (2022). The authors' effort deserves attentive analysis because, although it does not strictly defend a nudging perspective, it promises to overcome the liberty-autonomy conundrum while preserving the plurality of conceptions of the good in the process of policy justification. The spirit of this project is not far from how Thaler and Sunstein describe their own position: the ultimate judgment on preferences should be left to the agents themselves.

For Barnhill and Bonotti, eating policies tend to raise a whole host of ethical issues because food is a multifunctional object: "food is a resource necessary for sustenance and survival, and, as healthy eating efforts emphasize, food is a potential source of good (or bad) nutrition and health. But in addition to its role in promoting nutrition and physical health, food serves other personal and social functions" (Barnhill & Bonotti, 2022: 24). Eating "is central to virtually all kinds of human relationships and social groups", it is "linked to social and cultural identities", and it can also become a means for individuals to reach their aesthetic, ethical and political ends (Barnhill & Bonotti, 2022: 25). As Barnhill and colleagues have argued in a previous work, the discussion about "the informed or autonomous nature of food choices needs to be supplemented with a discussion of the value and disvalue of food experiences" (Barnhill et al., 2014: 188). These functions may come to clash with one another, while coexisting in the same person's hierarchy of ends: for instance, the consumption of fat or high-carb foods which in some cultures is associated with family gatherings and values is at odds with long-term plans of having a healthy life. "There are trade-offs involved in adopting healthier dietary patterns. This means that people may experience dilemmas surrounding healthy eating: people may have a range of ends to which eating is relevant, and they may not be able to simultaneously realize all those ends" (Barnhill & Bonotti, 2022: 30). In any case, Barnhill and Bonotti seem to privilege the "long-term life plans" of the individual as the lodestar for policy-making. Good health allows individuals to develop themselves overtime, thus constituting the essential background condition for the pursuance of their autonomously chosen ends. "Our view is that it is reasonable for public health policy-makers—as a general matter—to assume that many people's unhealthy dietary patterns are misaligned with their life plans, and to assume that making dietary patterns healthier would make many people better off by their own lights" (Barnhill & Bonotti, 2022: 36).

In general terms, they acknowledge that many instances of unhealthy food consumption are shaped by external factors, including limited availability and economic accessibility (such as in food deserts), aggressive marketing strategies, cultural and familial habits, as well as psychological and structural conditions like stress, precarious employment, and lack of time. In such cases, individual autonomy may be constrained or compromised, but it is not entirely absent. The authors reject the simplistic assumption that individuals make unhealthy choices merely because they are unaware of better alternatives or unwilling to choose them. They caution against the use of "non-voluntariness" as rhetorical cover for coercive or manipulative policy measures. Framing unhealthy eating as systematically irrational or involuntary risks supporting unwarranted forms of paternalism. Treating all unhealthy food choices as errors to be corrected or signs of manipulation reduces individuals to passive subjects in need of correction or re-education, rather than acknowledging them as morally autonomous agents and accepting that what constitutes a food item is strikingly personal and contextual (Borghini & Piras, 2021). While external influences certainly exist, they do not negate personal agency entirely. Ethical food policy, therefore, must resist the temptation to override individual autonomy in favor of ostensibly superior judgments about well-being, especially when such judgments are grounded in narrow or prescriptive understandings of rational behavior.

In Chapters 3 and 4 of their book, Barnhill and Bonotti develop a critique of the anti-paternalistic position in relation to healthy eating policies, starting from the well-known Millian objections and then transitioning to their contemporary interpretations. After discussing the various implications of the harm principle as formulated in *On Liberty*, Barnhill and Bonotti argue that "Mill would have accepted warning and persuasive healthy eating measures (e.g., food labels, including explicit and graphic ones), but not coercive measures such as limiting food portion sizes or the banning of certain foods. This does not mean, though, that Mill would not have accepted paternalistic healthy eating interventions *tout court*" (Barnhill & Bonotti, 2022: 98–99). In what follows, however, it is the whole liberal framework which is called into question. While autonomy should not be completely foregone as a moral value, the authors hold that reform efforts need not write a blank check to individual rationality in trying to cultivate opportunities for the flourishing of individuals. In spite of their earlier cautionary remarks, here Barnhill and Bonotti seem to take Thaler and Sunstein's assumption at face value: cognitive biases are a sufficient reason to accept the government as an assisting force in the practical articulation of people's life plans, most of all because the cognitive abilities of people are dulled by the choice environment they face. "The liberal ideal that governments should treat people as free and equal should not be construed as requiring governments to assume—contrary to ample empirical evidence—that individuals act rationally in pursuit of their conception of the good in This puts us in broad agreement with other work arguing that governments do not treat citizens disrespectfully when they accurately appraise citizens' rational abilities and design policies in light of predicted irrational behaviour" (Barnhill & Bonotti, 2022: 111–112).

But how can state intervention in the eating choices of citizens be justified? Barnhill and Bonotti argue that simply juxtaposing reasons for paternalism and for autonomy will not work. What is needed is a procedure which grants that collective decisions take into account and harmonize, as far as possible, individual conceptions of the good. The outcome will be accepted with equanimity, since it will be perceived as springing from a fair procedure. This is the essence of the *public reason* approach which was coined in John Rawls' *Political Liberalism* and has been given many different interpretations in contemporary political philosophy. Following the work of Vallier (2014), Barnhill and Bonotti (2022: 129) state that conceptions of public reason "vary with regard to which reasons should be allowed into the process of public justification" and "to what it takes for a policy or law to be justified or defeated by the reasons that are allowed into public justification". In a spectrum of options that ranges from complete anarchy/relativism to stricter constraints placed upon the admissible reasons (e.g., that they are widely shared at some level of abstraction), Barnhill and Bonotti take the middle ground, that is, the "accessibility" conception. The latter allows controversial reasons to be included in the debate, as long as they are formulated according to common "epistemic" and "evaluative standards". This means that "accessibility rules out as sources of public reason, e.g., those conceptions of health that rely on religious, supernatural, or folk explanations, whose epistemic grounds and methods of enquiry are widely contested and not accessible to those citizens who do not espouse such convictions" (Barnhill & Bonotti, 2022: 140).

The authors argue that this conception can be translated into a practical tool for policy-making and deliberation. They imagine the latter in the fashion of a questionnaire, to be submitted to members of expert boards, political representatives and common citizen—in some instances, Barnhill and Bonotti's sketch of deliberative structures resembles the idea of "mini publics" (Smith & Setälä, 2018), small local assemblies in which feedback can circulate more easily and in which the differential effect of policies can be discerned with higher accuracy. The questionnaire Barnhill and Bonotti envision seeks to assess the aims of policy proposals (whether they are only related to public health or they concern other areas of life), their potential side effects (e.g., enhancing discrimination for marginalized people with eating policies, such as those that prohibit buying soft drinks with food vouchers), and the balance of values they want to achieve (Barnhill & Bonotti, 2022: 188). If the feedback between experts and citizens is positive, the proposal will be publicly justified. Otherwise, it will be revised until an agreement is reached.

How effective is Barnhill and Bonotti's proposal in breaking the stalemate between paternalism and anti-paternalism? On the one hand, the public reason framework allows widening the criteria upon which policy-making is evaluated. While the debate around (libertarian) paternalism focuses only on the impact of policies on the subject's own good, public justification balances both "publicly-" and "privately-oriented" (Barry, 1965: 12–13) reform proposals. The need to protect individual liberty is thus mediated by more political concerns, merging deontological and consequentialist reasoning. On the other, public reason, bearing the trace of its contractarian origin, still emphasizes consent as the ultimate source of value. Moreover, Barnhill and Bonotti argue that this approach should not be confined to constitutional issues, but also extended to everyday political reform. This extension requires fine-tuned tools that, like the questionnaire they propose, are able to detect the trade-offs and the stratifications in individual preference rankings. The latter, as we have seen, are especially complex when it comes to eating matters.

It is not obvious that these two features blend well together. This difficulty is signaled by Barhill and Bonotti's conclusions: there is no assurance that, after all evaluations and reevaluations have been done, a policy will receive a clear enough justification. The authors often repeat that the objective of justification is "striking the right balance of values", but this end may just be too abstract for any procedure that, sooner or later, needs to produce a collective decision. Ultimately, there will always be a cleavage between input and output in collective action: some preferences *will* be overridden. On the other hand, if one focuses on the problem of how to respect individual conceptions of the good—like public reason promises to do—it is not easy to evade charges of paternalism. Barnhill and Bonotti assume, like Thaler and Sunstein do, that long-term health is a paramount concern for most people, and that paternalistic policies could be justified in helping them stick to this rational "system 2" (Kahneman, 2011) resolution against the everyday obstacles posed by cognitive biases. However, as we have seen in Sect. 2, this is a flawed argument: no fixed set of preferences can be taken as a definitive guide for policy-making.

Ultimately, Barnhill and Bonotti's book is useful because it points to a problem of consistency between theoretical approaches concerning food policies. If we endorse a perspective that places a big premium on consent and individual conceptions of the good, it will become increasingly difficult to find decisive reasons to subject many areas of people's lives to state intervention—especially if, like with eating, these areas are laden with moral and aesthetic values. In this respect, it is easier to fall back on Gerald Gaus' (1996) interpretation of public reason (explicitly rejected by Barnhill and Bonotti), whose radical pluralism justifies the liberal maxim "when in doubt, abstain" (De Jasay, 1997: 111). If that turns out to be the case, it will also become important to distinguish between different types of reasons — for example, those of experts, stakeholders, educators, or policy-makers, and laypeople (Borghini, 2023). On the contrary, if we want to frame the question of reform in purely political terms, we should accept the idea that individual autonomy and liberty will only play a subsidiary role. In this case, the moral content of public reason theories will be replaced by the attention given to coordination and collective action problems.

4 Food Ethics and the Justification of Nudging Policies

In the previous section, we distinguished between two ways of framing the problem of healthy eating within political theory. On the one hand, there is the paternalism/anti-paternalism divide, which focuses on the trade-off between individual autonomy and long-term personal health. In democratic contexts, there is broad agreement that individual conceptions of the good should be granted legitimacy, which may partly explain the appeal of libertarian paternalism. On the other hand, a more publicly oriented perspective shifts attention to the broader societal effects of dietary habits—on the economy, public services, and communal resources. BP is often regarded as the overarching ethical concern in public health policies that limit individual choice, but the debate is not always framed around how such limitations may affect public health outcomes. In this section, we focus on the latter perspective. Its advantage lies in avoiding the moral dimension of paternalism and instead treating healthy eating policies as potential solutions to coordination or collective action problems.

As public concern over the adverse health effects of poor diets has intensified, policy initiatives aimed at promoting healthier eating behaviors have also expanded. At various levels, governments have introduced or proposed a range of measures designed to shift dietary habits toward more nutritious choices. The European Union's food safety policy, for example, adopts a comprehensive 'farm to fork' approach aimed at ensuring that every stage of the food chain—from production and processing to distribution and consumption—meets strict safety and quality standards, while also promoting high standards of animal welfare, plant health, and environmental sustainability (e.g., Fiore et al., 2022;

Schebesta et al., 2020). In the United States, similar concerns, particularly the rising rates of overweight and obesity, have led to a variety of policy interventions, many of which have sparked significant ethical debate. Among the most contested are policies that limit the availability of certain foods, restrict access to specific products, or impose disincentives for their consumption (see Thow et al., 2014). Examples include proposed taxes on sugar-sweetened beverage, minimum nutritional standards for children's meals in fast-food establishments (such as the so-called Happy Meal ban), and zoning regulations aimed at reducing the density of fast-food outlets in certain neighborhoods (Hagenaars et al., 2021; Nelson & Banks, 2016; Wiley, 2013).

Unhealthy eating imposes various social costs, a paradigmatic example of which is the burden it places on publicly funded healthcare systems. When healthcare is collectively financed, widespread unhealthy consumption patterns can lead to a disproportionate use of shared resources by a segment of the population. As people engage in unhealthy eating, cases of preventable illnesses rise, thus increasing the demand for care. As a result, overall costs escalate, raising the question of how to finance the system or how to fairly distribute the resulting tax burden. This scenario resembles well-known models such as the prisoner's dilemma or the tragedy of the commons, where choices that appear rational from an individual perspective ultimately produce collectively irrational outcomes. Notably, free riding in this context need not stem from strategic intent; it may result from ignorance, limited foresight, or bounded rationality (for a summary of collective action dilemmas see Ostrom, 1990: ch. 1). Healthy eating policies, then, may be justified as a form of preventive intervention aimed at preserving collective welfare. Of course, such policy justifications are context-dependent and rely on institutional and cultural factors. They require a conditional 'if…then…' reasoning: if a health system is publicly financed, then unhealthy eating habits may generate externalities that justify regulatory intervention. Conversely, in a system based on private health insurance, responsibility tends to fall on the individual: if person A makes unhealthy choices at time t_0, it is not considered person B's responsibility to bear the cost of treatment at time t_1.

In this regard, we can follow the framework proposed by Guala and Mittone (2015), according to which nudges can be politically justified only when the behaviors they target generate intolerable externalities for the community. While Thaler and Sunstein ground nudging in the belief that individuals have true preferences that nudges help them achieve, Guala and Mittone argue that this assumption is often unjustified, as real-world preferences are unstable, context-dependent, and not easily identifiable. Since it is difficult to determine individuals' actual best interests and, as previously noted, there is a risk of conflating those interests with the preferences of policy-makers, the authors propose a political rather than purely welfarist justification for nudging. Justifying nudges based on externalities starts from the observation that behaviors shaped by cognitive biases can impose social costs, for instance, in cases of poor dietary choices, which place a burden on public systems. From this perspective, nudges are legitimate not because they enhance individual welfare, as public reason justifications would demonstrate, but because they help manage shared resources and reduce collective costs.

Naturally, the application of this "political" perspective need not be one-sided. As Guala and Mittone themselves admit, the notion of externality and the suitable solution are dependent on many cultural and political variables. For instance, the design and implementation of nudging policies could be left to agents other than the state, like private corporations. One possible approach to addressing the problem of externalities and determining which types of nudge policies are acceptable is to delegate this role to private institutions. In other words, we might envision a decentralized nudging landscape in which proposals emerge and are selected on a competitive basis. Such a framework could foster bottom-up solutions involving businesses as well as civil society organizations. However, the central question remains whether private actors can effectively internalize the externalities arising from individuals' biased decisions through decentralized nudging strategies, or whether such interventions must necessarily be carried out by public authorities. As Sunstein (2016) notes, the government, like the private sector, spontaneous orders and invisible hands, inevitably nudges. Several objections arise in response to this concern. One is that social responsibility may, at times, need to be imposed through political mechanisms, given that the primary objectives of private institutions are economic and profit-oriented. A prominent example is the phenomenon of greenwashing, used to attract environmentally conscious consumers without meaningful environmental commitment. Furthermore, critics may argue that private actors lack an inherent motivation to advance the public interest, particularly when nudging entails a degree of 'manipulation' influenced by vested interests. This is why it has been advocated a democratically controlled public policy nudging, which may serve to curb the power of private companies to nudge in opaque and unaccountable ways (Schmidt, 2017). Nonetheless, one might contend that allowing individual economic actors to define the scope of their social responsibility in relation to public issues could help resolve the normative challenge of identifying who is best positioned to implement nudge policies. This solution could be useful to overcome problems of authority justification and social responsibility: if the process of policy-making is not monopolized by any one actor, the perceived weight on the autonomy of individuals could be sensibly reduced. We might describe this as a 'market for social concerns'. Each company can choose to offer, indirectly and alongside its product, a specific set of moral principles. In turn, each consumer can decide to reward certain of these value packages through their purchasing decisions. Moreover, this solution could enhance the cost-effectiveness properties of nudging, since constant experimentation allows for a better filtering out of inefficient solutions.

5 Final Remarks

This chapter has explored the ethical and political complexities surrounding Behavioral Paternalism (BP), particularly as it applies to food policy. The debate faced a number of important questions: first and foremost, to what extent is it possible, in a pluralistic society, to design policies that do not implicitly impose a hierarchy of values? While proponents of BP present it as a libertarian-friendly tool for improving individual welfare, we have argued that it often relies on contested interpretations of behavioral data and reintroduces normative assumptions under the guise of an alleged neutrality. In doing so, it risks subordinating plural and context-dependent individual preferences to externally defined standards of rationality or well-being. The deliberative model proposed by Barnhill and Bonotti offers an important corrective by seeking legitimacy through public reason. However, its reliance on procedural consensus may prove insufficient in contexts, like food policy, where values are deeply personal and culturally embedded. Indeed, the various positions examined—from critiques of 'benevolent' paternalism to the deliberative proposal advanced by Barnhill and Bonotti, and the systemic reading of coordination problems—all demonstrate that any attempt at regulation rests, more or less explicitly, on a particular vision of what truly matters for individuals and society. Ultimately, the challenge lies in developing institutional frameworks that balance collective concerns with respect for individual autonomy, while maintaining transparency about the normative choices embedded in public policy. Even strategies that present themselves as 'neutral' (or at least 'non-paternalistic') inevitably incorporate normative judgments. The crucial question then becomes: is it truly possible, in a pluralistic society, to design public policies that do not impose—even implicitly—a hierarchy of ends? Or must we acknowledge that every political intervention, even when justified by public reason or aimed at addressing externalities, inevitably entails a degree of interference with individual choices? This question appears destined to remain open. Precisely for this reason, it becomes essential to develop theoretical and practical tools capable of making the normative assumptions of policy choices transparent, so that they can be more effectively subjected to public debate and critical revision. The tension between autonomy and public health will never be definitively resolved. Yet awareness of the normative underpinnings of public policies can help us design interventions that are more transparent, flexible, and just. In this sense, the future of food ethics will depend on our ability to combine political pragmatism with moral sensitivity—recognizing that, in the realm of everyday choices, there are no perfectly neutral solutions, but only ever-negotiable balances between freedom, individual responsibility, and justice. Addressing this challenge is essential not only for the future of food ethics, but also for the broader legitimacy of behavioral interventions in democratic societies.

References

Aird, R. (2023). A puzzle of epistemic paternalism. *Philosophical Psychology, 36*(5), 1011–1029. https://doi.org/10.1080/09515089.2022.2146490

Barnhill, A., & Bonotti, M. (2022). *Healthy eating policy and political philosophy: A public reason approach.* Oxford University Press.

Barnhill, A., & Civita, N. (2020). Ethics of healthy eating. In H. Meiselman (Ed.), *Handbook of eating and drinking* (pp. 1173–1195). Springer. https://doi.org/10.1007/978-3-030-14504-0_91

Barnhill, A., King, K. F., Kass, N., & Faden, R. (2014). The value of unhealthy eating and the ethics of healthy eating policies. *Kennedy Institute of Ethics Journal, 24*(3), 187–217. https://doi.org/10.1353/ken.2014.0021

Barry, B. (1965). *Political argument*. Routledge & Kegan Paul.

Boettke, P. J. (2000). Why culture matters: Economics, politics, and the imprint of history. In P. J. Boettke (Ed.), *Calculation and coordination: Essays on socialism and transitional political economy* (1st ed.). Routledge. https://doi.org/10.4324/9780203469682

Borghini, A. (2023). Healthy foods, healthy diets, and healthy eating: Beyond ethics and political philosophy. *Food. Ethics, 8*(14). https://doi.org/10.1007/s41055-023-00124-8

Borghini, A., & Piras, N. (2021). On interpreting something as food. *Food Ethics, 6*, 1–10.

Buchanan, J. M. (1949). The pure theory of government finance: A suggested approach. *Journal of Political Economy, 57*(6), 496–505. https://doi.org/10.1086/256880

Congiu, L., & Moscati, I. (2022). A review of nudges: Definitions, justifications, effectiveness. *Journal of Economic Surveys, 36*(1), 188–213. https://doi.org/10.1111/joes.12453

Conly, S. (2013). Coercive paternalism in health care: Against freedom of choice. *Public Health Ethics, 6*(3), 241–245. https://doi.org/10.1093/phe/pht025

De Jasay, A. (1997). *Against politics: On government, anarchy, and order.* Routledge.

Dold, M. (2023). Endogenous preferences: A challenge to constitutional political economy's normative foundation? *Constitutional Political Economy, 36*, 424–443. https://doi.org/10.1007/s10602-023-09417-w

Dold, M., Harper, D., Rajagopalan, S., & Whitman, G. (2024). Process, rationality and human wellbeing. *Behavioural Public Policy*, 1–10. https://doi.org/10.1017/bpp.2024.60

Entwistle, T. (2021). Why nudge sometimes fails: Fatalism and the problem of behaviour change. *Policy & Politics, 49*(1), 87–103. https://doi.org/10.1332/030557320X15832072208458

Fiore, M., Sauvée, L., & Wiśniewska-Paluszak, J. (2022). Opportunities and challenges of EU farm-to-fork strategy. *International Food and Agribusiness Management Review, 25*(5), 703–707. http://dx.doi.org/10.22434/IFAMR2022.x001

Gaus, G. (1996). *Justificatory liberalism: An essay in epistemology and political theory*. Oxford University Press.

Gigerenzer, G. (2004). Fast and frugal heuristics: The tool of bounded rationality. In D. Koehler & N. Harvey (Eds.), *Handbook of judgment and decision making* (pp. 62–88). Blackwell Publishing. https://psycnet.apa.org/doi/10.1002/9780470752937.ch4

Gigerenzer, G. (2015). On the supposed evidence for libertarian paternalism. *Review of Philosophy and Psychology, 6*(3), 361–383. https://doi.org/10.1007/s13164-015-0248-1

Gigerenzer, G., & Gaissmaier, W. (2011). Heuristic decision making. *Annual Review of Psychology, 62*, 451–482. https://doi.org/10.1146/annurev-psych-120709-145346

Grüne-Yanoff, T. (2012). Old wine in new casks: Libertarian paternalism still violates liberal principles. *Social Choice and Welfare, 38*(4), 635–645. https://doi.org/10.1007/s00355-011-0636-0

Grüne-Yanoff, T., & Hertwig, R. (2016). Nudge versus boost: How coherent are policy and theory? *Minds and Machines, 26*(1), 149–183. https://doi.org/10.1007/s11023-015-9367-9

Guala, F., & Mittone, L. (2015). A political justification of nudging. *Review of Philosophy and Psychology, 6*, 385–395. https://doi.org/10.1007/s13164-015-0241-8

Hagenaars, L. L., Jeurissen, P. P. T., Klazinga, N. S., Listl, S., & Jevdjevic, M. (2021). Effectiveness and policy determinants of sugar-sweetened beverage taxes. *Journal of Dental Research, 100*(13), 1444–1451. https://doi.org/10.1177/00220345211014463

Hausman, D. M., & Welch, B. (2010). Debate: To nudge or not to nudge. *Journal of Political Philosophy, 18*(1), 123–136. https://doi.org/10.1111/j.1467-9760.2009.00351.x

Hayek, F. A. (1937). Economics and knowledge. *Economica, 4*(13), 33–54. https://doi.org/10.2307/2548786

Hayek, F. A. (2008). In B. Caldwell (Ed.), *The road to serfdom. Text and documents: The definitive edition.* Routledge.

Kahneman, D. (2003). Maps of bounded rationality: Psychology for behavioral economics. *American Economic Review, 93*(5), 1449–1475. https://doi.org/10.1257/000282803322655392

Kahneman, D. (2011). *Thinking, fast and slow.* Farrar, Straus and Giroux.

Kuyer, P., & Gordijn, B. (2023). Nudge in perspective: A systematic literature review on the ethical issues with nudging. *Rationality and Society, 35*(2), 191–230. https://doi.org/10.1177/10434631231155005

Nelson, B., & Banks, K. (2016). Super-sized strategies for improved health: Does reducing the density of fast food restaurants matter? In C. Bosso (Ed.), *Feeding cities: Improving local food access, security, and resilience* (pp. 55–72). Routledge. https://doi.org/10.4324/9781315627137

Oliver, A. (2023). *A political economy of Behavioral public policy.* Cambridge University Press.

Ostrom, E. (1990). *Governing the commons: The evolution of institutions for collective action.* Cambridge University Press.

Polanyi, M. (2015). *Personal knowledge: Towards a post-critical philosophy.* The University of Chicago Press.

Rizzo, M. J. (2016). The four pillars of behavioral paternalism. In S. Abdukadirov (Ed.), *Nudge theory in action: Behavioral Design in Policy and Markets* (pp. 37–63). Springer International Publishing. https://doi.org/10.1007/978-3-319-31319-1_3

Rizzo, M. J., & Whitman, G. (2019). *Escaping paternalism: Rationality, behavioral economics, and public policy.* Cambridge University Press.

Schebesta, H., Bernaz, N., & Macchi, C. (2020). The European Union farm to fork strategy: Sustainability and responsible business in the food supply chain. *European Food and Feed Law Review, 15*(5), 420–427.

Schmidt, A. T. (2017). The power to nudge. *American Political Science Review, 111*(2), 404–417. https://doi.org/10.1017/S0003055417000028

Simon, R. A. (1976). From substantive to procedural rationality. In T. J. Kastelein, S. K. Kuipers, W. A. Nijenhuis, & G. R. Wagenaar (Eds.), *25 years of economic theory: Retrospect and Prospect* (pp. 65–86). Martinus Nijhoff. https://doi.org/10.1007/978-1-4613-4367-7_6

Smith, G., & Setälä, M. (2018). Mini-publics and deliberative democracy. In A. Bächtiger, J. S. Dryzek, J. Mansbridge, & M. Warren (Eds.), *The Oxford handbook of deliberative democracy* (pp. 300–314). Oxford University Press. https://doi.org/10.1093/oxfordhb/9780198747369.013.27

Storr, V. H., & John, A. (2020). *Cultural considerations within Austrian economics*. Cambridge University Press.

Sugden, R. (2018). *The Community of Advantage: A behavioural economist's defence of the market*. Oxford University Press.

Sunstein, C. R. (2016). *The ethics of influence: Government in the age of behavioral science*. Cambridge University Press.

Thaler, R. H. (2016). Behavioral economics: Past, present, and future. *American Economic Review, 106*(7), 1577–1600. https://doi.org/10.1257/aer.106.7.1577

Thaler, R. H., & Sunstein, C. R. (2003). Libertarian paternalism. *American Economic Review, 93*(2), 175–179. https://doi.org/10.1257/000282803321947001

Thaler, R. H., & Sunstein, C. R. (2008). *Nudge: Improving decisions about health, wealth, and happiness*. Yale University Press.

Thow, A. M., Downs, S., & Jan, S. (2014). A systematic review of the effectiveness of food taxes and subsidies to improve diets: Understanding the recent evidence. *Nutrition Reviews, 72*(9), 551–565. https://doi.org/10.1111/nure.12123

Trout, J. D. (2005). Paternalism and cognitive bias. *Law and Philosophy, 24*, 393–434. https://doi.org/0.1007/s10982-004-8197-3

Turner, S. (2024). Epistemic coercion. *Epistemology & Philosophy of Science, 61*(3), 21–38. https://doi.org/10.5840/eps202461337

Tversky, A., & Kahneman, D. (1974). Judgement under uncertainty: Heuristics and biases. *Science, 185*(4157), 1124–1131.

Vallier, K. (2014). *Liberal politics and public faith: Beyond separation*. Routledge.

Viale, R. (2022). *Nudging*. MIT Press.

Wiley, L. F. (2013). Sugary drinks, happy meals, social norms, and the law: The normative impact of product configuration bans. *Connecticut Law Review, 46*(5), 1877–1881.

Zappia, C. (1996). The notion of private information in a modern perspective: A reappraisal of Hayek's contribution. *The European Journal of the History of Economic Thought, 3*(1), 107–131. https://doi.org/10.1080/10427719600000006

For a Relational Well-Being in Food Advertising: Beyond Healthism and Foodporn

Veronica Neri and Silvia Dadà

1 Introduction

In recent years, particularly in the wake of the Covid-19 pandemic, interest in healthy lifestyles and balanced nutrition has grown exponentially—not only among public policymakers and the general public, but also in media discourse. *Healthy living* has acquired increasing appeal, both in the domain of food and in the broader context of fitness and personal well-being (Andersen et al., 2021; Krogager & Leer, 2024).

Within such evolving cultural landscape, two complementary currents appear to emerge. On the one hand, healthism can be understood as a lifestyle oriented towards self-care, where *substance* (well-being) is pursued through the cultivation of *form* (physical and mental fitness).

V. Neri (✉) · S. Dadà
Department of Civilisation and Forms of Knowledge, University of Pisa, Pisa, Italy
e-mail: veronica.neri@unipi.it

S. Dadà
e-mail: silvia.dada@unipi.it

F. Bruno et al. (eds.), *Healthcare and Food*,
https://doi.org/10.1007/978-981-95-5899-5_6

On the other hand, the phenomenon of foodporn reverses such logic: here, the aestheticized *form* of food is privileged and even fetishized, often standing in for *substance* itself. These two models, while seemingly opposed, offer complementary visions of food consumption. Both are grounded in a subject-object dynamic that isolates the individual from the broader social, cultural, and environmental contexts.

Within such conceptual framework, we see blogs, social media platforms, and advertising strategies flourish that actively seek to shape how individuals conceptualize eating and, more specifically, healthy eating. Both influencers and everyday users increasingly curate narratives of healthy living through aestheticized presentations of nutritious food, references to nutraceutical practices, and attention to body care (David & Allard, 2022).

Our analysis centres on a particular strand of the *foodporn* phenomenon—one that does not merely celebrate the sensual or aesthetic dimension of food but rather integrates it into the relational and ethical framework of nourishment. Such approach entwines with the broader question of human flourishing, echoing the classical ideal expressed by Seneca: *mens sana in corpore sano.*[1]

What we aim to argue is that food imagery, especially as mediated by digital platforms, is a new form of self-representation—one that need not be confined to individualist or hedonistic paradigms. On the contrary, the visual stimulation of appetite and pleasure can function as a medium of ethical significance, fostering a culture of care, hospitality, and shared well-being. In this light, *foodporn* may serve as a catalyst for promoting *relational well-being*, understood as an ethical condition grounded in attentiveness to others, communal eating practices, and mutual recognition.

Such reframing suggests that the dynamic of self-isolation—often exacerbated by neoliberal modes of consumption and self-optimization—can be reoriented. When *healthism* and *foodporn* are made to talk with each other, they may embrace an aesthetics of

[1] L.A. Seneca (1917–1925), *Epistulae morales ad Lucilium—Lettera 15* (R.M. Gummere, Transl.). London: W. Heinemann, about the importance of leading a life based on the philosophical theories of a wise man while protecting the physical wellbeing of the individual (*corpus*).

the everyday that is ethically generative. Through digital media, ludic engagement, and the visual culture of food, one may cultivate not only healthier lifestyles but also a deeper, more embodied understanding of well-being—relationally conceived, and not merely as an individual possession. Such a perspective aligns with philosophical traditions that conceive of the self as constituted through intersubjective and material relations, rather than as an autonomous, self-contained entity.

2 From Healthism to Mass-Mediated Food

We will now turn to a brief conceptual clarification of *healthism*, before exploring how it intersects with mass-mediated food advertising, and particularly its emphasis on the visual and sensory appeal of food—rich textures, vibrant colours, and indulgent presentations.

In its origin, *healthism* can be understood as a cultural and behavioural paradigm, encompassing normative frameworks and embodied practices aimed at safeguarding health and optimizing the individual's physical and psychological well-being. Initially conceived of as a "lifestyle that prioritizes health and fitness over anything else", such notion has gradually acquired a more value-laden connotation.

Over time, it has come to denote an attitude characterized by an intense, at times excessive, preoccupation with one's health. This shows as a continuous effort to adhere to strict regimes of hygiene, nutrition, and body regulation, often framed as moral imperatives. In this sense, healthism reflects not merely a concern for biological functioning, but also an ethical posture grounded in self-surveillance and personal responsibility.

From a philosophical standpoint, this shift aligns with broader biopolitical logics, according to a Foucauldian theory, whereby care for the self becomes intertwined with disciplinary rules. Health is no longer simply a state of being but becomes an aesthetic and ethical project, turning the body into a site of both self-expression and social control. In its most pervasive form, healthism participates in the moralization of lifestyle, linking personal virtue to corporeal discipline and placing the burden of well-being squarely on the individual.

Such framework becomes particularly significant when viewed in relation to food advertising and digital food culture, where the pursuit of health often intersects with aesthetic consumption. As we shall see, the interplay between healthism and media-driven representations of food opens a space for rethinking the ethics of eating, embodiment, and relational well-being.[2]

According to the thinking of Irving Zola, who theorized the concept in 1977, it is part of medicalization, which he firmly criticized (Conrad, 1992; Zola, 1972, 1977). In his opinion, a paradigm shift has taken place and "[h]ealth itself became not merely the means to some larger end but the end in itself, no longer one of the essential pillars of the good life but the very definition of what is the good life" (Zola, 1977: 51). For the economist Robert Crawford, who addressed this concept a few years later, personal dedication to health is conceived not primarily as a response to illness but as a pathway to well-being—achievable through the cultivation of a proper lifestyle rather than through conventional medical intervention. Healthism, from such perspective, emerges as an autonomous phenomenon, grounded in an *expansive* understanding of medicine; one that is not necessarily opposed to traditional clinical practices, yet operates alongside or even beyond them. It is a mode of self-governance, whereby the subject takes responsibility for the regulation of their own physical and psychological condition, often outside institutional frameworks (Crawford, 1980)·

For both, the 'medicalisation' of everyday life also extends to lifestyles. Crawford, in particular, defined healthism as "the preoccupation with health as a primary – often the primary – focus for the definition and the achievement of well-being; a goal which is to be attained primarily through the modification of lifestyles, with or without therapeutic help" (Crawford, 1980: 368).

Thus, practices such as fitness routines and specialized diets come to weave together sport, aesthetics, and medicine.

Today, these are increasingly integrated with wellness apps—now widely used—which monitor and support dietary habits, real-time

[2] Cf. Headword *Healthism* in the Collins Online Dictionary; Headword *Salutismo* in Voc. Treccani online.

metabolic data, and physical training. These technologies act as a form of virtual personal coaching: while not replacing the expertise of medical professionals, they offer motivational support by providing users with data that track their progress towards specific goals, while detailing milestones and outcomes in a quasi-narrative format.

The phenomenon of *healthy living* is reinforced by pervasive cultural pressure, driven by media and advertising, which capitalize simultaneously on the desire to be healthy and high-performing, and on the modern compulsion for control. This dual impulse may be interpreted as a reaction to the uncertainty and unpredictability of the external world: in the face of systemic instability, individuals retreat into the domain of the body, perceived as one of the few remaining spaces of personal agency. Health becomes the object of a hyper-rationalized and individualized form of supervision.

In this light, *healthism* takes the shape of a regime of self-surveillance, operating as a moral obligation towards oneself. From a philosophical standpoint, extreme forms of healthism can be read as a distorted appropriation of Foucault's ethics of care of the self, an ethics that, while initially conceived of as a form of self-cultivation and autonomy, is now subsumed into disciplinary structures aimed at the normalization of the body. In this context, healthism is not merely a cultural phenomenon, but a symptom of deeper transformations in the relationship among subjectivity, embodiment, media technologies, and social norms.

Health-oriented lifestyles are also increasingly intertwined with public health programmes aimed at discouraging high-risk behaviours such as smoking, obesity, and physical inactivity. Such dynamics has given rise to what is often referred to as "coercive healthism", whereby the state actively promotes the stigmatization of practices deemed harmful to health (Skrabanek, 1994). In such cases, health becomes a moral and political imperative, framed not only as a right, but also as a civic duty. The promotion of well-being thus serves as a criterion for *"good" citizenship*, reinforcing a normative ideal of bodily discipline and self-management.

Within such a framework, food advertising may act as a vehicle for such health discourses, contributing to the subject's well-being through nutritional messaging. Social campaigns promoted by the state, non-profit organizations, or even individuals exemplify how media can support public health goals by shaping consumption habits in ethically charged ways.

However, the contemporary media landscape points to a parallel and seemingly contradictory phenomenon: foodporn. At first glance, foodporn seems to subvert the logic of healthism. It entails the *aestheticisation* of food for its own sake, a spectacular, often hyper-stylized representation of food designed to captivate audiences and elicit visual pleasure rather than promote nutritional value. In this context, consumption becomes primarily visual instead of dietary, oriented towards desire and entertainment (Spence et al., 2016; Taylor & Keating, 2018).

In what follows, we will explore the origins of foodporn and consider how it might, paradoxically, be redirected towards an ethics of *relational health*. Beyond its superficial indulgence, foodporn has the potential to be reinterpreted not merely as a form of visual consumption, but as a cultural tool for rethinking care, relationality, and shared embodiment through food. Yet, this phenomenon warrants closer examination.

3 Foodporn for Well-Being

The foodporn phenomenon is quite recent. It was first mentioned by Roland Barthes in his 1957 collection, Mythologies, who defined it as 'that which offers fantasies to those who cannot afford to cook certain meals' (Barthes, 1957: 78; McBride, 2010). After two decades, in 1977, journalist Alexander Cockburn used the term gastro-porn in the *New York Review of Books.* Two years later, in 1979, Michael Jacobson used the term 'food pornography' in the newsletter of the Center for Science in the Public Interest, in connection with certain representations of food that were sensationally far beyond what food should be (Cockburn, 1977). The term later gained prominence through the work of feminist writer Rosalind Coward, who, in the early 1980s, reflected on the sensual representation of food in popular culture and the affective allure it generates in the viewer (Coward, 1984: 103). In her seminal work *Female Desire: Women's Sexuality Today*, Coward conceptualized "food pornography" as a shift from the notion of food as a gift—a gesture of care or relational offering—to food as an object of aesthetic pleasure and visual consumption. Such transformation, she suggested, marks a deeper cultural reconfiguration of desire, in which the ethics of nourishment are displaced by an economy of spectacle and superficial gratification. This shift from food as care to food as spectacle calls for a critical rethinking of how food practices and representations might instead cultivate empathy, connection, and ethical engagement.

Coward, in fact, wrote that:

> But it is only the unfortunate readers of the slimming magazines who are supposed to use the pictures as a substitute for the real thing. While other forms of food photography are meant to stimulate the desire to prepare and eat the food, for the slimmers it is a matter of feasting the eyes only. (Coward, 1984: 102–103)

And then:

> The purpose of these photos is to show perfect dishes out of context, namely from the kitchen and the preparation process [...] Just as we know that glamorous advertising models are not really what they appear to be, so we know just as well that preparing a meal takes many hours in which a lot of things get dirty and messy. (Coward, 1984: 107)

Coward also emphasized that foodporn primarily targets a female audience, aiming to evoke a subtle sense of guilt. It often showcases visually appealing dishes that stand in stark contrast to prevailing social imperatives surrounding body image and thinness. In this regard, foodporn becomes a site of internal moral tension: it invites indulgence through aesthetic pleasure while simultaneously reinforcing disciplinary rules concerning bodily self-regulation.

A different genre of foodporn, however, seeks to reconcile such tension by making low-calorie or "healthy" foods visually enticing. Such subcategory attempts to align the aesthetic enjoyment of food with the pursuit of a desirable physique, thereby shifting the experience from one marked by guilt to one oriented towards self-affirmation and self-presentation. The underlying message becomes: consuming beautiful food leads to becoming beautiful. Such logic inspires a form of aesthetic self-promotion, where the act of eating is entwined with the cultivation of an idealized self-image.

Moreover, a growing fascination with highly stylized representations of food can elicit a sense of unattainability, reinforcing the divide between the viewer and the idealized culinary product. Such visual culture of food often intersects with trends such as *show cooking* and *food design*. The latter refers not only to the design of dish presentations but to a broader aesthetic orchestration of culinary experiences as well: from the configuration of communal dining spaces and culinary technologies to the artistic layout of table settings. At its core, food design reflects a reimagining of the relationship between human beings and food, one that privileges aesthetic sensibility as a key medium of interaction, meaning-making, and shared experience.

Culinary techniques aimed at producing appetizing dishes are often designed to elicit an instinctive form of pleasure—the pleasure of eating *well*. But what does *well* mean in this context? Within the framework of foodporn, it frequently denotes a form of consumption oriented towards visual gratification: eating with the eyes, satisfying the gaze, even at the expense of nutritional value or concerns about food waste. Here, the act of eating is aestheticized, and the sensuous appeal of the dish often overrides its material or ethical substance.

Such dynamics evokes, albeit in a different guise, the classical ideal of καλὸς κἀγαθός, the inseparable unity of the beautiful and the good. In this context, food becomes the contemporary stage on which this ancient ideal is performed, albeit often with an emphasis on *form* over *function*, and appearance over sustenance.[3]

As Deborah Lupton has argued for over three decades, food, beyond its biological necessity, acts as a cultural and social symbol, central to the construction of collective identity. It is not merely a reflection of individual preferences or personal taste; it is embedded within broader social, moral, and even religious codes. Food, in this sense, operates

[3] To foodporn we can associate, as Perullo suggests, the aesthetics of Zen cuisine and the experiments of conceptual chefs and up to food design, to achieve the pleasure of eating well by combining ethics and aesthetics. See Mangano (2014), Munari (2003), Perullo (2014: 27 ff.), and Vozelgang (2009).

as both a mirror and a mediator: it reveals personal choices while simultaneously inscribing the individual within a network of shared meanings, expectations, and values (Lupton, 1996, 2020). Foodporn occurs in multiple forms, all grounded in a shared aesthetic principle: the exuberant aestheticization of food that is not necessarily healthy, but intensely sensual and indulgent. At its core lies the logic of *desire* and the *anticipation* of consumption, where the pleasure is mediated primarily by visual engagement. This aestheticization of food may also intersect with discourses of *healthism*, especially when the act of "eating well" is seen to have tangible effects on one's physical appearance and bodily performance. In such cases, the underlying normative framework is a compromise between aesthetic pleasure and nutritional value, adjusted to the specific needs and ideals of one's own body.

It is the latter configuration—where foodporn converges with health-conscious practices to reconcile beauty and bodily well-being—that our analysis will now turn to.[4]

The representation of food has been profoundly reshaped by food designers, food stylists, and the narrative techniques of media celebrities who teach us how to prepare dishes that are often aesthetically unattainable, step by step, turning cooking into a spectacle of perfection. Within such dynamics, the dimension of care and authentic sharing in the preparation of food becomes subordinate to its transformation into a primarily visual and symbolic object of consumption, rather than one rooted in material nourishment or relational practice.

And yet, if, as Ludwig Feuerbach famously maintained, "man is what he eats", then feeding oneself on pleasurable and healthful food responds to the intertwined demands of both physical and psychological well-being. The shift from food in its natural state, raw and untouched, to its cooked, cultural, and socially mediated form has increasingly become both the object and subject of contemporary food advertising. These

[4] Parallel to foodporn, the phenomenon of gastro-anomy, defined by Claude Fischler as an overabundance of discourses on food without rules, also arises. Franchi, in turn, pointed to the 'crisis of the relationship between the modern individual and food and the rise of the dominance of a serial diet determined by industrial production and speed', inspired by food multinationals and mass society'. See Fischler (1990), Franchi (2009, 2015), and Pollan (2008).

media representations strategically play on such duality, i.e. staging food as both a natural substance and a cultural performance.

The antinomies "nature/culture" and "raw/cooked" highlight not only food's function as sustenance, but also its manipulability, its ability to be transformed into a multiplicity of forms and meanings (Lévy-Strauss, 1964: 1 ff.). Culinary techniques, in this symbolic framework, mark the passage from the *natural state* of rawness to the *cultural state* of cooked food, making room for conviviality and relational engagement. As Claude Lévi-Strauss insightfully observed, "the cuisine of a society unconsciously translates its structure—or even reveals, without knowing it, its contradictions" (Lévy-Strauss, 1990: 445).

Indeed, the contemporary visual culture of food, with its dazzling colours and exuberant abundance spilling from serving platters, becomes a mirror of a society that is both materially opulent and deeply contradictory. On the one hand, there is an obsession with food as a source of aesthetic gratification; on the other, a drive towards limitation and restraint, focused on quality and quantity at the service of a disciplined, healthy, and "fit" body. Both trends seem to operate within a broader hedonistic ethics, centred on self-pleasure and self-affirmation through the perfection of lifestyle practices.[5]

4 What Kind of Well-Being?

In contemporary food advertising, two dominant narratives shape how we perceive our relationship with food: the health-oriented narrative and the *foodporn* aesthetics.

The health-focused narrative promotes an ideal of self-care through nutrition. It emphasizes the consumption of natural, wholesome foods as a pathway to achieving physical, psychological, and emotional balance. Within such a framework, the individual is portrayed as the central agent—someone who, through disciplined eating and lifestyle choices, attains a desirable state of well-being. Visual representations often feature

[5] N. Perullo, *Filosofia del cibo*, cit., pos.1101.

slim, smiling individuals engaged in physical activity, reinforcing the association between healthy eating, personal success, and happiness.

In contrast, the *foodporn* narrative shifts the focus from the subject to the object—food itself. Here, the emphasis lies on the visual and sensory appeal of food: rich textures, vibrant colours, and indulgent presentations. The food is not necessarily healthy, but it is aesthetically irresistible. Such narrative prioritizes emotional and psychological gratification, often side-lining concerns about nutrition or physical health. The viewer is invited to experience pleasure through the image alone, making the act of consumption secondary to the visual enjoyment.

Despite their differences, both narratives share a common structure: they frame the relationship with food as a binary interaction between an isolated subject (the consumer) and an object (the food). Such framing excludes other actors and dimensions that are essential to a more holistic understanding of food and well-being.

To critically assess the implications of such narratives, we can turn to the concept of *food well-being* as defined by Blok et al., who describe it as "a positive psychological, physical, emotional, and social relationship with food at both the individual and societal levels" (Block et al., 2011). Compared to this definition, the advertising narratives feel reductive. The health-focused model attempts to integrate psychological, physical, and emotional dimensions, but often isolates the individual from their social and environmental context. The *foodporn* model, meanwhile, emphasizes psychological and emotional satisfaction—primarily through aesthetic pleasure—while neglecting physical health and broader social implications.

As Setiffi (2011) insightfully observed, the advertising language around food products often reduces well-being to a static, commodified concept, something attainable through purchase. Such narrative promotes two contrasting yet interconnected body models: the active body, typical of the fitness consumer, who engages in self-improvement through disciplined consumption; and the passive body, which seeks pleasure through relaxing, effortless experiences. However, the line between these two is blurred. It is the very nature of the well-being commodity that draws both types of bodies into the same cycle of consumption, reinforcing a market-driven vision of health and pleasure. What is particularly lacking in both narratives is the collective and contextual dimension of food well-being. Eating is not merely a solitary act of consumption; it is embedded in cultural, familial, and environmental contexts that shape our experiences and perceptions of food. The setting in which food is consumed—whether communal or isolated, sustainable or exploitative—plays a significant role in shaping well-being. Moreover, such narratives often ignore the cultural, social, and emotional bonds that food and shared meals help to construct.

This brings us to the concept of *relational well-being* (White, 2017, 2023; Wissing, 2014), which offers a more expansive and inclusive framework for understanding food and well-being. Relational well-being emphasizes the importance of social connections, shared experiences, and the environments in which such interactions occur. It moves beyond the subject-object binary and situates food practices within a broader social fabric.

Atkinson (2013) provided a compelling rethinking of well-being through a relational lens. She argues that well-being is not an individual possession but something that emerges from assemblages of relationships among people, places, material objects, and intangible elements such as atmosphere. From such perspective, well-being is profoundly situated and relational, arising from the "movement and clusterings of affect" that occur at specific intersections of time and space. It is not a static attribute of individuals but a dynamic, collective experience.

Social theories of the self as relational further support such perspective. These theories posit that relationships precede subjectivity, meaning that our sense of self is formed through our interactions with others. From this standpoint, community well-being is not simply the sum of individual well-beings but a shared state of "being well together" (Atkinson et al., 2020). So, well-being is not a personal possession but something that emerges through meaningful connections with others.

Translating this into the realm of food means rethinking the self in relation—not as an isolated consumer, but as someone embedded in a web of social, cultural, and ecological ties. This shift expands the notion of care beyond the solipsistic focus on individual health or pleasure. Care becomes the cornerstone of a new narrative, in which food plays a qualitatively rich role, situated within the relationships and contexts in which it is consumed.

A valuable contribution to such perspective came from Nicola Perullo (2022) (see also Pelluchon, 2019), who suggested that we should focus less on the specific contents of food and more on the dispositions that emerge from the ways food is offered and consumed. As opposed to an ontology that classifies food based solely on its nutritional or aesthetic properties, Perullo proposed a relational and modal approach—a "dietetics of care" grounded in sensitivity and attentiveness to what we eat and the situations in which food is experienced.

Similarly, Adriano Fabris (2024) emphasized that the goal should not be limited to monitoring and controlling one's physical form. Rather, it should involve cultivating a respectful, balanced relationship that acknowledges the multiple connections in which every living being is involved. This includes not only interpersonal relationships but ethical and ecological considerations too.

To move closer to a more holistic and inclusive understanding of food well-being, it is essential that we reframe our narratives. This means recognizing food not just as a means to an end—whether health or pleasure—but as a medium through which relationships are built and sustained. It involves acknowledging the importance of context: the spaces in which we eat, the people we eat with, and the systems that produce and distribute our food (Shotwell, 2021).

These dimensions of what we might call *relational food well-being* can be meaningfully encapsulated in the concept of *care*. Food is a powerful mediator of care for and attention to others (Furst, 2017). Feeding is, in fact, one of the earliest expressions of care—beginning in the womb and continuing through various social practices (Dadà, 2021; Ruddick, 1989). From family meals to communal gatherings, food plays a central role in how we express affection, support, and connection.

Significant life events are often marked by shared meals, where food takes on symbolic meanings. Reconnecting food to this relational and social function allows us to move beyond the individualistic focus of health-centric narratives and the objectifying, aestheticized lens of *food-porn*. Instead, it invites us to see food as part of a broader web of relationships—emotional, cultural, and ethical—that shape our well-being and our sense of belonging.

5 Food as Care in Advertising

Embracing a relational approach to food well-being challenges the prevalent individualistic models and opens up new possibilities for thinking about food as a shared, meaningful, and transformative experience. It invites us to consider not only what we eat, but how, where, and with whom we eat—and how these dimensions shape our collective well-being.

While advertising continues to shape the prevalent perceptions of food and well-being, it also offers an opportunity for critical reflection. By challenging the individualistic assumptions embedded in such narratives and embracing a relational approach, we can begin to construct more inclusive, equitable, and meaningful understandings of what it means to eat well and live well—together.

Looking beyond the prevalent narratives of health-focused eating and *foodporn*, we find that the idea of food as care is not entirely missing from advertising. Particularly in Italian advertising, food is often portrayed as a symbol of emotional bonds, social connection, and joyful sharing.

Roland Barthes famously analysed this in his semiotic reading of a Panzani (Barthes, 1998) pasta advertisement, highlighting how the connotative language of both text and image evokes a rich network of meanings. The arrangement of products and the use of warm colours suggest grocery shopping, Italian identity, and the authenticity of home-made meals. Altogether, the imagery conjures up the warmth of home and the maternal care embedded in everyday routines. Even the mesh bag with the products subtly recalls the shape of a womb, reinforcing the theme of nourishment and protection (Codeluppi, 2010).

From the 1980s onwards, under the creative direction of Gavino Sanna (1988), Barilla adopted a new branding strategy centred on family, domesticity, and emotional values.

Prior to this, pasta advertising focused mainly on product quality and practical use (de Martini, 2017). As Semprini and Musso observed, Sanna's approach shifted towards utopian messaging, promoting "feminine values opposed to masculine ones, care opposed to commerce" (Semprini & Musso, 2010: 53). Through dichotomies such as male/female, public work/private home, and rationality/emotion, Barilla emphasized the link between food—specifically pasta—and care. In this sense, we can identify an early form of *relational food well-being*.

With the launch of the famous slogan *"Where there's Barilla, there's home"*, Barilla positioned itself at the very heart of domestic life. In doing so, it entered the collective imagination through the syllogism: *"Pasta = Home, Pasta = Barilla, therefore Barilla = Home"* (Semprini & Musso, 2010: 32).

During the pandemic, amid global health uncertainty, many advertisements shifted their focus towards social well-being and both individual and collective physical and mental health. Central to such campaigns was the home, portrayed as a place of care, safety, and responsibility. This emphasis marked a second form of *relational food well-being*, with food becoming a vehicle for messages of social solidarity that extended beyond close family ties. In this context, food advertising contributed to what Giorgino described as a "culture of responsibility" (Giorgino, 2020). In these messages, food was often symbolic or even absent, as the spotlight turned to community values and the call for unity. In that dramatic historical moment, these ideals took precedence over market-driven concerns, highlighting the role of food communication in fostering collective resilience.

So, food advertising offers more than just the prevalent narratives of health-consciousness and foodporn. It also draws on values such as care, responsibility, and solidarity to construct an imaginative framework in which food is embedded within meaningful relational networks. These campaigns expand the notion of well-being by highlighting the emotional and social dimensions that food can foster. However, this narrative is not without its challenges. One concern is that it may diminish the role of pleasure—an essential aspect of taste and central to the experience of food. By shifting the focus away from the product itself, the sensory and hedonic qualities of food risk being overlooked or deemed secondary. A more holistic view of well-being should integrate such dimension, recognizing pleasure and taste as vital components of the eating experience.

Another significant concern is the recurring association between care and femininity. As highlighted in discussions on the ethics of care (Held, 2005; Tronto, 1995), such perspective can reinforce and legitimize traditional gender roles, particularly those that assign caregiving, cooking, and domestic responsibilities to women. Many advertisements keep depicting the family in a conventional framework, portraying women as the "angel in the house" (Papakristo, 2013), thereby perpetuating outdated stereotypes instead of challenging them. Additionally, such narratives often reinforce national stereotypes. The strong link between food, pasta, and Italian identity can lead to caricatured representations of Italy—oversimplified and, at times, offensive. Advertising frequently relies on stereotypical imagery and simplified portrayals of reality, which can unintentionally promote discriminatory views.

In response to such trend, several brands, including those in the food industry, have begun to introduce more diverse and unconventional family representations (multiracial families, same-sex families, single-parent families, etc.) (Boero, 2018). Such efforts aim to foster a more inclusive and dynamic understanding of family, care, and the emotional value of social bonds, which go beyond static and exclusionary ideals.

In conclusion, both health-oriented and foodporn advertising models promote individualistic notions of well-being, overlooking the broader social, cultural, and environmental dimensions of food practices. Such approaches reduce food to either a tool for self-optimization or to a source of visual and sensory pleasure, neglecting its deeper role in building community, shaping identity, and creating shared meaning.

An alternative to such models is found in food advertisements that embrace the concept of *relational well-being as care*. In such campaigns—like those by Barilla—food is portrayed as a catalyst for social bonds and caring practices. However, even this model carries potential risks, such as abstracting food away from pleasure or reinforcing stereotypical representations of care, identity, and relationships. Aware of such limitations, food advertising can evolve by reimagining its language and imagery towards a more inclusive vision of well-being as care—one that harmoniously integrates happiness and pleasure with health, shared responsibility, and emotional connection.

References

Andersen, T., Byrne, D. V., & Wang, Q. J. (2021). How Digital Food Affects Our Analog Lives: The Impact of Food Photography on Healthy Eating Behavior. *Frontiers in Psychology, 12*, 12.

Atkinson, S. (2013). Beyond Components of Well-Being: The Effects of Relational and Situated Assemblage. *Topoi, 32*, 137–144.

Atkinson, S., Bagnall, A. M., Corcoran, R., et al. (2020). Being Well Together: Individual Subjective and Community Well-Being. *Journal of Happiness Studies, 21*, 1903–1921.

Barthes, R. (1957). *Mythologies*. The Noonday Press.

Barthes, R. (1998). The Rhetoric of the Image. In N. Mirzoeff (Ed.), *The Visual Culture Reader* (pp. 135–138). Routledge.

Block, L. G., Grier, S. A., Childers, T. L., Davis, B., Ebert, J. E. J., Kumanyika, S., Laczniak, R. N., Machin, J. E., Motley, C. M., Peracchio, L., Pettigrew, S., Scott, M., & Bieshaar, M. N. G. G. (2011). From Nutrients to Nurturance: A Conceptual Introduction to Food Well-Being. *Journal of Public Policy & Marketing, 30*(1), 5–13. https://doi.org/10.1509/jppm.30.1.5

Boero, M. (2018). *La famiglia della pubblicità. Stereotipi, ruoli, identità*. Franco Angeli.

Cockburn, A. (1977). Gastro-Porn. *New York Review of Books.*

Codeluppi, V. (2010). *Persuasi e felici? Come interpretare i messaggi della pubblicità*. Carocci.

Conrad, P. (1992). Medicalization and Social Control. *Annual Review of Sociology, 18*, 209–232.

Coward, R. (1984). *Female Desire: Women's Sexuality Today*. Paladin.

Crawford, R. (1980). Healthism and the Medicalization of Everyday Life. *International Journal of Health Services, 10*(3), 365–388.

Dadà, S. (2021). *Maternità e alterità*. ETS.

David, G., & Allard, L. (2022). An Anatomy of the Meal Gaze. In E. J. H. Contois & Z. Kish (Eds.), *Food Instagram: Identity, Influence, and Negotiation* (pp. 65–93). University of Illinois Press.
de Martini, A. (2017). *Brand Narrative Strategies: il segreto dell'onda.* Franco Angeli.
Fabris, A. (2024). *Etica delle Relazioni Alimentari.* Springer.
Fischler, C. (1990). *L'homnivore: le goût, la cuisine et le corps.* Odile Jacob.
Franchi, M. (2015). La nuova cultura alimentare: dalla gastro-anomia alla diet-etica. *Atti dell'Accademia dei Georgofili,* VIII, vol. 12, II, 3.
Franchi, M. (Ed.) (2009). *Il cibo flessibile. Nuovi comportamenti di consumo.* Carocci.
Furst, M. (2017). Care and Nutrition: Ethical Issues: Exploring the Moral Nexus Between Caring and Eating Through Natural History, Anthropology and the Ethics of Care. *Rel.: Beyond Anthropocentrism, 5,* 103.
Giorgino, F. (2020). La pubblicità al tempo del Coronavirus, "*AIS" 2020/16*, 206–207.
Held, V. (2005). *Ethics of Care, Personal, Political, and Global*. Oxford University Press.
Krogager, S. G. S., & Leer, J. (2024). Foodporn 2.0? Definitions, Challenges, and Potentials of an Elusive Concept. *Journal of Aesthetics & Culture, 16*(1).
Lévy-Strauss, C. (1964). *The Raw and the Cooked* (J. Weightman & D. Weightman, Trans.). Plon
Lévy-Strauss, C. (1990). *The Origin of Table Manners* (first edition 1968). University of Chicago Press. It. Trans. (1971), *Le origini delle buone maniere.* II Saggiatore.
Lupton, D. (1996). *Food, the Body and the Self*. Sage Publication.
Lupton, D. (2020). Carnivalesque Food Videos: Excess, Gender and Affect on YouTube. In D. Lupton & Z. Feldman (Eds.), *Digital Food Cultures* (pp. 35–49). Routledge.
Mangano, D. (2014). *Che cos'è il food design.* Carocci.
McBride, A. (2010). Foodporn. *Gastronomica: The Journal of Food and Culture, 10,* 38–46.
Munari, B. (2003). *Good design* (first edition 1963). Carraini Editore.
Papakristo, P. C. (2013). *Il volto delle sirene: storia della figura femminile nella pubblicità italiana.* Aras.
Pelluchon, C. (2019). *Nourishment: A Philosophy of the Political Body.* Bloomsbury.
Perullo, N. (2014). *Cibo, estetica e arte. Convergenze tra filosofia, semiotica e storia.* Edizioni ETS

Perullo, N. (2022). Toward a Relational Aesthetics as Dietetics of Care: On Eating Meat. *Teoria. Rivista di Filosofia, 42*(1), 133–148.
Pollan, M. (2008). *Il dilemma dell'onnivoro.* Adelphi.
Ruddick, S. (1989). *Maternal Thinking: Toward a Politics of Peace.* Beacon Press.
Sanna, G. (1988). *Le uova di Woody Allen. Guida arbitraria ai misteri e ai piaceri della pubblicità.* Bompiani.
Semprini, A., & Musso, P. (2010). Dare un senso alla marca. In M. Lombardi (Ed.), *Il dolce tuono. Marca e pubblicità nel terzo millennio.* Franco Angeli.
Setiffi, F. (2011). La mercificazione del benessere postmoderno. In D. Secondulfo (Ed.), *Sociologia del benessere. La religione laica della borghesia.* Franco Angeli.
Shotwell, A. (2021). Flourishing Is Mutual: Relational Ontologies, Mutual Aid, and Eating. *Feminist Philosophy Quarterly, 7*(3). https://doi.org/10.5206/fpq/2021.3.10850
Skrabanek, P. (1994), *The Death of Humane Medicine and the Rise of Coercive Healthism.* Social Affairs Unit.
Spence, C., Okajima, K., Cheok, A. D., Petit, O., & Michel, C. (2016). Eating with Our Eyes: From Visual Hunger to Digital Satiation. *Brain and Cognition, 110*, 53–63.
Taylor, N., & Keating, M. (2018). Contemporary Food Imagery: Foodporn and Other Visual Trends. *Communication Research & Practice, 4*(3), 307–323.
Tronto, J. C. (1995). *Moral Boundaries.* Routledge.
Vogelzang, M. (2009). *Eat Love. Food Concepts by an Eating Designer*. Bis.
White, S. C. (2017). Relational Well-Being: Re-Centring the Politics of Happiness, Policy and the Self. *Policy & Politics, 45*(2), 121–136.
White, S. C. (2023). Relational Well-being. In F. Maggino (Ed.), *Encyclopaedia of Quality of Life and Well-being Research.* Springer.
Wissing, M. P. (2014). Meaning and Relational Well-Being: A Reflection on the State of the Art and a Way Forward. *Journal of Psychology in Africa, 24*(1), 115–121.
Zola, I. K. (1972). Medicine as an Institution of Social Control. *Sociological Review, 20*(4), 487–504.
Zola, I. K. (1977). Healthism and Disabling Medicalization. In I. Illich, I. K. Zola, J. McKnight, J. Caplan, & H. Shaiken (Eds.), *Disabling Professions* (pp. 41–67). Marion Boyars.

"Eat When You Are Hungry": Ethics of Eating/Food from the Perspective of the Buddhist-Christian Dialogue

Seung Chul Kim

> What goes into someone's mouth does not defile them, but what comes out of their mouth, that is what defiles them.
> Matthew 15:11
> The intention and the words of the buddhas and ancestors are like everyday tea and rice.
> Furong Daokai (芙蓉道楷 1043-1118)

1 Eating/Food as a Religious and Theological Issue

We are what and how we eat, and it is we who do the eating. As is said, we can tell who you are if you tell us what you eat (Brillat-Savarin, 1970: 13). The issue of eating/food is intrinsically linked to human beings'

S. C. Kim (✉)
Nanzan Institute for Religion and Culture, Nagoya, Japan
e-mail: sechkim@gmail.com

F. Bruno et al. (eds.), *Healthcare and Food*,
https://doi.org/10.1007/978-981-95-5899-5_7

self-understanding, which is carried out through their relationships with themselves, with the world in which they think they find themselves, and with what they believe provides both humans and the world with their ultimate foundation. Thus, the ethical awareness of eating/food emerges with the understanding that eating fosters a relationship between the eater and the eaten, because what and how we eat inevitably connects us to other living things, such as animals and plants. That relationship is further broadened to encompass the traditions and eating habits of people from different religions and cultures, as well as the environment of the Earth in which we produce food.

When the ethics of eating/food matter, we often find that such discussions occur on the premise that ethics has to do with finding the place where people are allowed and accustomed to living. The term ethics is derived from *ethos*, meaning "an accustomed place or habitation," from which the following connotations are derived: "customs," "attitudes," "moods," as well as the "boundaries" between such human habitats and the unknown beyond them. Furthermore, *ethos* also refers to the distinction between wild animals and domestic animals (Incandela, 1996: 59–60).

In short, ethics is regarded as a problem about setting the proper boundary between humans, nature, and the divine, whatever it means. The harsh controversies surrounding "Dolly the cloned sheep," sparked by the birth of a sheep through cloning in 1996, provide a good example of how debates on ethics revolve around the questions of where and who can set the boundary that should not be transgressed. Is it God or human beings? The clash between two American theologians, Paul Ramsey and Joseph Fletcher, who have made significant contributions to the birth of the discipline of bioethics, can be summarized as an uncompromising collision of two catchphrases: "Man ought not to play God" and "Let us play God." At the same time, the controversies surrounding the term "playing God" raise the question of what we could or should "play" in a world where no "God" is supposed to be, such as in a society pervaded by the Buddhist understanding of reality (Kim, 2016: 63–70).

In this sense, it is understandable that the *ethics* of eating/food were initially developed in a close relation with biotechnology and bioethics. Ben Mepham, who was then the director of the Center for Applied

Bioethics at the University of Nottingham, UK, and who is considered to have coined the term of "Food Ethics," made it clear that his concerns are "with a branch of social ethics which is relevant to public policy, and which in turn will guide the implementation of necessary regulations on the employment of biotechnology in food production" (Mepham, 1996: 104). Many of the ethical controversies we have had so far regarding eating/food have been aimed at finding the proper boundary between what we may eat and what we may not, such as the controversy pro and contra of eating meat, the alternative proposal of veganism or vegetarianism, for example, as a substitute for meat eating, and organic farming as an alternative to factory farming.

As the close relationship between bioethics and "food ethics" shows, the ethical argument about eating/food presupposes, consciously or unconsciously, that it prompts us to consider the religious foundations of our being. Recent studies on the history of religion reveal that the theme of eating/food played an indispensable role in building an exclusive identity of any religious community by selecting and rejecting specific foods. Just as the *kashrut* in Judaism and *halal* in Islam show, favoring or avoiding a specific food determines the exclusive identity of a particular religious community. In this sense, we can agree with the opinion that "recipes for cooking could be a kind of ritual manual that can tell us more about the complex things we call religion, and how they have been cooked and how food will be served in the future" (Nam, 2021: 240).

In this essay, I want to try to answer the question of what kind of ethics of eating/food is required when the different religions and cultures encounter each other so closely that we must admit the fact that "purely intrareligious problems – themes that are relevant for one religion only – have ceased to exist" (Van Bragt, 2014: 44). For that, I would like to discuss how the issue of eating/food is understood and practiced in Christianity and Zen Buddhism.

2 Biblical and Christian Wisdom on Eating/Food

The issue of eating/food in the Bible, especially in the teachings and behaviors of Jesus and His disciples in Early Christianity, reveals some critical moments that could be meaningful in our age of crisis and conflict: the crisis in the human-nature relationship and the conflict among religions and ideologies. The taboos listed in Leviticus 11 in the Old Testament became the model for the extensive and systematic Jewish dietary laws (Cha, 2008: 99–135). This rule had a significant impact on Jewish nutritional practices to the point that, even in the New Testament era, non-Jews who enjoyed pork were considered unclean by this standard. However, as suggested by the episode of Cornelius (Acts 10:9–16), the new perspective that repulsive animals, according to Leviticus, could be made clean and thus edible through divine power served as a symbolic message supporting the legitimacy of missionary work among the Gentiles: "Do not call anything impure that God has made clean."

The mission begins by crossing the boundaries drawn by traditional taboos regarding specific foods considered "impure." The mission is to be understood as an ongoing process of decoding and depatterning "the code" of the particular food associated with a religious tradition (Douglas, 1971: 61–81).

Jesus also declared that all foods are clean (Mark 7:19). He criticized the Jewish dietary laws, maintaining that it is not what goes into the mouth that defiles a person, but what comes out of the mouth (Mark 7:20). Jesus did not adhere to the traditional Jewish eating/food description, which was the reason that he was criticized as "a glutton and a drunkard, a friend of tax collectors and sinners" (Matthew 11:19). Instead, Jesus broke with the customs of self-proclaimed religious people and associated with sinners, opening up the exclusive table where a specific group of people shared and divided certain religious privileges among themselves. This was a deliberate act that demonstrated the universality of the Kingdom of God, without boundaries. By applying the principles of purity and impurity, which were previously used to food regulations, to human society, it became an alternative political expression aimed at transforming the self-perpetuating system that sought to solidify barriers of exclusion and discrimination. Jesus removed the label of "sinner" imposed on those on the margins of society and restored the essence of life to them. Furthermore, this act served to proclaim the creative principle that food, as a gift of God's grace, should be distributed without discrimination to all people. Jesus transcended the discriminated line between the pure and the impure, which can be an ethic beyond ethics as an awareness of drawing a line.

For Jesus, eating/food touches, far beyond the question of what we may eat and what we may not, the ground of human beings' life, as it has been argued that the Hebrew word for human life (*nepes*) has the same meaning as food, and that the word for God's covenant (*berit*) is etymologically derived from the word meaning "to eat" (*barah*) (Jenks, 1992: 250–254). "In fact, the theological dynamics of meals presented in the New Testament appear to have served as an important catalyst for dismantling existing norms that had become firmly fossilized and opening up new horizons (Cha, 2008: 101).

Paul also stated, on the one hand, that since all food comes from God, there is no problem in eating it with thanksgiving (1 Corinthians 10:30; 1 Timothy 4:4). On the other hand, Paul recommended a self-restriction of eating everything to care for those whose faith is weak and cannot eat all, and to restrain oneself from blaming those who eat everything: "One person's faith allows them to eat anything, but another, whose faith is weak, eats only vegetables. The one who eats everything must not treat with contempt the one who does not, and the one who does not eat everything must not judge the one who does, for God has accepted them" (Romans 14:2–3). The same self-restraint is recommended in matters of eating food that has been sacrificed to idols. Some people are aware that the idol is nothing, so the food sacrificed to it has no power to influence their faith. However, some people with weak faith and knowledge are concerned that consuming such defiled food will erode their faith. Paul's admonitions are mainly pointed to those who think their faith is mature: "Be careful, however, that the exercise of your rights does not become a stumbling block to the weak" (1 Corinthians 8:9). So, Paul continues: "Do not destroy the work of God for the sake of food. All food is clean, but it is wrong for a person to eat anything that causes someone else to stumble. It is better not to eat meat or drink wine or to do anything else that will cause your brother or sister to fall" (Romans 14:20–21).

What is essential in the issue of eating/food for Jesus, and for Paul, too, is that they demand us to be free from attachment or discrimination toward a specific food. In short, the Christian tradition of eating/food did not draw a sharp line between what one may eat and what one may not eat, just as we can find in the Jewish tradition. Instead, as we have seen in Paul's attitude toward the issue of eating/food above, Christian faith taught freedom with a consideration for the weak in their faith. Even though the history of Christianity and the history of monastic life show us various understandings of eating/food, especially regarding the question of eating meat, we can say roughly that the spirit of the freedom of Christians, as seen in Paul and later in Martin Luther during the age of Reformation, allowed Christians a rather broad choice list of eating/food. To put the same thing the other way around, Christians are asked to get over the discriminatory exclusiveness regarding the question of what we may eat and what we may not.

3 Zen Buddhism on Eating/Food

What can we learn from Buddhism about eating/food? When discussing Buddhist attitudes toward eating/food, we must first acknowledge that there has been no uniform discipline or habit in Buddhism regarding which foods are permitted to be eaten and which are not. When it comes to Buddhism and the ethics of eating/food, there has been diversity, just as there have been various Buddhist traditions throughout different times and regions. Obviously, we could already say that, from the very Early Buddhism, there has existed "a very strong anti-hunting and anti-animal killing agenda," and veganism was considered as "an appropriate dietary regime to reach purity and moral perfection" (Tarocco et al., 2024: 262–263). However, in detail, there has been a variety of eating/food habits. For example, Buddhists in Thailand, where the Theravada Buddhist tradition has prevailed, do not hesitate to eat meat except for some particular animals like elephants and horses, which are perceived as sacred, lions and tigers, which might attack wandering monks, or dogs and snakes, which are considered to be impure and poisonous. Above all, the regulation of eating/food is conducted according to the spirit of detaching from any selfish behavior, meaning "the egoistic attitude implied in expressing an intention, as choosing a specific food for satisfying a personal physical desire (it does not matter if it is a vegan, vegetarian, or animal food option)" (Tarocco et al., 2024: 260–261).

Unlike Hinduism, Buddhism did not ban eating meat itself. Buddha himself once immersed himself in the ascetic practices, which were a standard form in India at the time, including fasting and eating only one grain of rice per day. However, he was unable to attain enlightenment through these practices, so he abandoned asceticism, regained his strength by eating milk porridge offered by a village girl, and then attained enlightenment while meditating under a bodhi tree, becoming the Buddha, the Enlightened One (Yorizumi, 2009: 301).

It cannot be said that Buddhism completely denies all desires, including appetites. It is acceptable in Buddhism to satisfy the minimum appetite necessary to maintain physical and mental health and continue spiritual practice. What is unacceptable is excessive eating driven by desire or being overly particular about food and seeking out delicious flavors. In other words, the basic Buddhist attitude toward food is to consume the minimum amount necessary without attachment to it (Yorizumi, 2009: 301). The issue of eating/food is also to be thought in relation to the Buddhist ontology. When the minimum requirement is exceeded, the desire for food is negated as a defilement. Defilements are attachments, and attachments are impurities that hinder spiritual practice.

Furthermore, Buddhism did not follow the discriminative rules prohibiting eating together with the untouchables, as was described in the caste system of Brahmanism in India. According to the *Mahāparinibbāna Sutta*, which contains the end of Gautama Buddha's life, he became ill from food poisoning after eating mushrooms that a man named Cunda Kammāraputta had offered. Cunda is said to have been a metalworker, and under the caste system of the time, that job belonged to a lower caste. Despite this, the Buddha accepted the offerings of someone from such a low caste. As recorded in the same sutra, he also showed compassion to Cunda, ensuring he would not regret having caused his death through Cunda's offerings. The following story reveals that Buddha was not reluctant to eat something donated by the then-current outcast people, which highlights one of the most essential themes to remember when discussing the issue of eating/food in Buddhism (Vajira & Story, 1964: 32).

After eating what was offered by Cunda, Buddha experienced deadly pain and fell into a dreadful sickness, which led to his death. And before his death, Buddha left the following admonitions to his most beloved disciple, Ānanda;

> Then the Blessed One spoke to the Venerable Ānanda, saying: "It may come to pass, Ānanda, that someone will cause remorse to Cunda the metalworker, saying: 'It is no gain to you, friend Cunda, but a loss, that it was from you the Tathāgata took his last alms meal, and then came to his end.' Then, Ānanda, the remorse of Cunda should be dispelled after this manner: 'It is a gain to you, friend Cunda, a blessing that the Tathāgata took his last alms meal from you, and then came to his end". (Vaijira & Story, 1964: 36)

As stated, Buddhism, from its inception, has denied fasting as a spiritual practice and acknowledged the necessity of consuming the bare minimum amount of food. By all means, Buddhism prohibits drinking liquor through its Five Precepts, which prohibit killing, stealing, sexual misconduct, lying, and intoxication. Drinking alcohol itself was not regarded as a sin but was forbidden due to its bad results. The reason that eating meat itself was not banned in Indian Buddhism came from the thought that monks should eat without discrimination, whatever was donated to them. Such a spirit of respecting those who offer food as an offering was carried forward in Mahayana Buddhism, which can be inferred from the fact that monks' behavior of begging food was not only for the sake of monks themselves but also for ordinary people who cannot be monks and live in the secular world. Begging and offerings were ways provided for ordinary people to attain Buddhist ideals. *Bhikshu* (monk) and *Bhikshuni* (nun) meant initially "beggars." When it was time to eat, ascetic monks would beg for food and eat whatever lay believers offered them without being picky. And "this practice of begging is stipulated in the twelve ascetic practices of early Buddhism. Ascetic practice is a transcription of the Sanskrit word "*dhūta*," which originally means "to cast off," and refers to the practice of casting off the defilements of the mind and abandoning greed for food, clothing, and shelter in order to devote oneself to ascetic practices" (Yorizumi, 2009: 301).

Chinese Buddhism differed from Indian Buddhism in that the former, from the beginning, had a community living in a temple built with the support of the state, so they did not need to rely on begging for food. The focus of the ethics of eating/food shifted from the controversy of eating meat to the community and the ordinary life of the monks, which ultimately gave rise to Zen Buddhism, regarded as a Buddhist tradition most deeply rooted in Chinese culture.

In Zen Buddhism, all aspects of daily life, including farming and household chores, were regarded as Buddhist practices. These practices were called "*samu*" (作務, working in the temple) and were considered to be as crucial as *zazen* meditation. A Chinese Zen monk named Baizhang Huaihai (百丈懷海 720–814) is said to have established a set of rules for Zen monks, known as the *Baizhang Zen Monastic Regulations* (百丈清規). (We can compare it to the Rule of St. Benedict.) "If one does not work for a day, one should not eat for a day (一日不作一日不食). In light of those considerations, Guishan Lingyou (潙山靈祐 771–853), a prominent Zen master in the Chinese Tang dynasty, reminds his monastic audience of its indebtedness to others. He strongly criticizes monks who abuse the privileges bestowed on them by failing to approach their religious vocation conscientiously: "How can you declare 'I am a monk' as soon as you receive the monastic precepts? The lay donors provide the daily necessities and the monastery's permanent property. Without understanding or properly considering where they come from, you [mistakenly] assume they are supplied in a natural way, as a matter of fact" (Poceski, 2006: 23). Such a spirit of respecting the intention of the food donors is vividly alive in the meditation ceremony that monks repeatedly perform before eating. Monks recite the following *Five Contemplations* (*kokan no ge* 五観の偈):

> First, regarding how great an effort [brought us this food], we consider where it has come from.
> Second, we reflect on whether our virtue and practice are worthy of receiving this offering.
> Third, to protect the mind, abandoning our mistakes from greed, hate, and delusion is essential.
> Fourth, truly this good medicine is for healing our fragile bodies.
> Fifth, now we receive this food for the sake of accomplishing Buddha's Way. (Dōgen, 1996: 92)

It is clear why monks cite Five Reflections before eating. Wanting to be free from the attachment to food, they accept it with gratitude to the donor, the cook, and above all, to all living things whose lives were taken so that they could be eaten. Eating is rather a sorrowful behavior of confessing one's absolute weakness and sin, which means we could not live without depriving the lives of other living beings. The banquet table is then a confessional booth for the sacrament of penance.

The writings on cooking and eating by Dōgen (道元 1200–1253), who represents the Sōtō school of Zen in Japan, inherited those traditions of Buddhist monastic regulations for the everyday life of monks in the temple. *Instructions for the Cook* (*Tenzokyōkun* 典座教訓) is an instruction on how and with what state of mind a monk should prepare food in a temple, while *The Dharma for Taking Food* (*Fushukuhanpō* 赴粥飯法) teaches a monk how and with what state of mind a monk should eat.

Whereas the ascetic tradition in Christianity and also in Buddhism in common had often tended to view the body "as different from and less than the soul," which had yielded "the mortification of the body, the strong deemphasis, even denial, of it," and while we could find a similar attitude to it in the Buddhist tradition, Zen monastic tradition reveals a relatively flexible attitude toward eating and drinking (Henry, 2001: 53–55). In "*Instructions for the Cook,*" Dōgen emphasizes that cooking, as a daily task in the temple, is equivalent to seeking the Buddhist dharma, the truth. There, kitchen work is a form of spiritual cultivation almost equal to meditation, as we read in his book:

> Since ancient times, masters with Way-seeking mind, lofty people who had awakened their hearts, were appointed to this job. After all, isn't this the single color of diligently engaging in the Way? If you do not have the mind of the Way, then all of this hard work is meaningless and not beneficial. The *Zen'en Shingi* says, 'You must put to work the mind of the Way, offering appropriate variety [in the food served] so that the community can feel satisfied and at ease. (Dōgen, 1996a: 33)

Cooking is a very way of dharma seeking, which demands a *tenzo*, a cook-monk, to abandon any kind of discrimination about food. There should not be a rich and poor food. Here, we can find the old Buddhist tradition of begging, which instructs the begging monk to receive whatever is offered by the people with gratitude.

> Cooking so-called rich, creamy food is not necessarily superior, cooking plain vegetable soup is not necessarily inferior. When you are given plain vegetables to prepare, you must treat them the same as rich, creamy food, with straightforward mind, sincere mind, and pure mind. The reason is that when they converge in the pure great ocean assembly of Buddha Dharma, you recognize neither rich, creamy tastes nor the taste of plain vegetables, but only the flavor of the one great ocean. Furthermore, in developing the buds of the Way and nurturing the womb of sages, rich cream and simple vegetables are the same, not different. There is an old saying that a monk's mouth is like an oven. We should understand this. Reflect that simple vegetables can nurture the womb of sages and develop the buds of the Way. Do not see them as lowly or worthless. A guiding teacher of humans and celestial beings benefits them with plain vegetables. (Dōgen, 1996a: 43–44)

Tenzo's work of cooking is to be done as a practice of no-mind. He deals with the materials given to him for cooking as if he treats the ultimate truth, *dharma*, which demands, for its part, to break through the nothingness of the mind. Dharma itself is, of course, nothingness, too. Thus, we can say that the monk-cook, the materials for cooking, and the cooked as a result of cooking are the same in that they have no self-identities in themselves (Dōgen, 1996a: 44).

Just cooking is a practice, so is eating. In his book, *The Dharma for Taking Food*, Dōgen quotes phrases from the *Vimalakirti Sutra* saing "If you can remain the same with food, all dharmas also remain the same; if all dharmas are the same, then also with food you will remain the same," Dōgen then added the following explanation: "Just let dharma be the same as food, and let food be the same as dharma. For this reason, if dharmas are the dharma nature, then food also is the dharma nature. If the dharma is suchness, food also is suchness. If the dharma is the single mind, food also is the single mind. If the dharma is bodhi, food also is bodhi. They are named the same and their significance is the same, so it is said that they are the same" (Dōgen, 1996b: 83).

What does this "same" mean? Dōgen replied that this "same" is not the sameness of parity or equality, but the sameness of awakening to the true sameness [*anuttara Samyak sambodhi*]. "Awakening to the true sameness is the ultimate identity [of all the suchnesses] from beginning to end. The suchness of the ultimate identity from beginning to end is the genuine form of all dharmas, which only a buddha together with a buddha can exhaustively penetrate. Therefore, food is the dharma of all dharmas, which only a buddha together with a buddha exhaustively penetrate. Just at such a time, there are the genuine marks, nature, substance, power, function, causes, and conditions. For this reason, dharma is itself food, food is itself dharma. This dharma is what is received and used by all buddhas in the past and future. This food is the fulfillment that is the joy of dharma and the delight of meditation" (Dōgen, 1996b: 83–84).

The phrase that dharma is food, and food is dharma, means that food and dharma are nothing but "the self here and now" (Furuyama, 2007: 5). They are the emergence of the self. We remember here the Buddhist ontology. Everything exists in dependent origination (*pratītya-samutpāda*), and therefore, nothing has its everlasting foundation in itself. But this "nothing," *śūnyatā*, does not have its foundation in itself, either. "Nothing" is nothing and empty, too. Just as we must be liberated from the attachment to the things, so must we abandon the attachment to *śūnyatā*, too. In Zen, such a Buddhist "ontology" or "logic" is expressed in a straightforward yet paradoxical manner that there is no need even to be awakened because every behavior emerges from the true nature of a human being, the true self, as Mazu said:

> It is in contrast to ignorance that one speaks of awakening. Since originally there is no ignorance, awakening also need not be established. All living beings have since limitless eons ago been abiding in the *samādhi* of the Dharma-nature. While they are in the *samādhi* of the Dharma-nature, they wear their clothes, eat their food, talk, and respond to things. As they make use of the six senses, all their activity is the Dharma-nature. Because of not knowing how to return to the source, they follow names and seek forms. That gives rise to confused emotions and falsehood, thereby creating all kinds of karma. If one were able within a single instant to illuminate within, then the whole essence is the holy mind. (Poceski, 2007: 218)

Already in the masterpiece of his Zen understanding, *Treasury of the True Dharma Eye* (正法眼蔵*Shōbōgenzō*), Dōgen stressed that eating in ordinary life is "the same" as the "extraordinary matter" in Zen practice, which means "sitting alone on Daxiong Peak." Being busy moving around to prepare meals is equivalent to sitting alone on top of a high mountain meditating, because to forget oneself by being indulged in working is tantamount to being selfless through meditation:

> In the house of the buddhas and ancestors, there is always "the extraordinary matter": it is "sitting alone on *Daxiong Peak*." Even to encounter here "let this fellow sit there" — this is also "the extraordinary matter." Going further, there is something even more extraordinary than that: it is "*The Jinci pātra bowl has moved to Tiantong to have rice*." Each and every instance of "the extraordinary matter" is "having rice." Thus, "sitting alone on Daxiong Peak" — this is "having rice". (Dōgen, 2023: 295)

As mentioned above, one of the characteristics of Zen Buddhism is its emphasis on the everydayness and non-extraordinary nature. Thus, having rice as a habit in daily life is no different from a heroic behavior of sitting alone on top of a mountain for meditation. An anecdote on eating/food from Huaihai tells us the typical Zen Buddhist way of understanding eating/food:

> A Vinaya master named Yüan once came and asked:

'Do you make efforts in your practice of the Way, Master?'
M: 'Yes, I do.'
Q: 'How?'
M: 'When hungry, I eat; when tired, I sleep.'
Q: 'And does everybody make the same efforts as you do, Master?'
M: 'Not in the same way.'
Q: 'Why not?'
M: 'When they are eating, they think of a hundred kinds of necessities, and when they are going to sleep they ponder over affairs of a thousand different kinds. That is how they differ from me.' At this, the Vinaya Master was silenced". (Blofeld, 1962: 95–96).

Zen Buddhism always teaches that when you are hungry, you eat; when you are sleepy, you sleep (飢来喫飯、困来即眠), which represents that the ordinary mind is the truth (平常心是道) (Koga: 76). *The Faith-mind maxim* (Xin-xin Ming 信心銘), composed by Seng Can (僧璨 645–667), tells us:

The perfect Way is not difficult;
It only avoids discrimination.
If only there is no love or hate,
Completely clean and clear is it. (Cleary, 1999: 123; Cf. Koga, 1991: 173–174)

In his Book, *Treasury of the True Dharma Eye*, Dōgen himself emphasizes the ordinary works we repeat every day, without even noticing the meaning behind those works. For example, in Ch. 59, "Everyday Matters" (*kajō* 家常), Dōgen says as follows:

Within the house of the buddhas and ancestors, tea and rice are everyday matters. The meaning of this tea and rice has long been passed on and is realized even now. Therefore, the way of life of the tea and rice of the buddhas and ancestors has come down to us. Thus, we should clearly maintain this: that "the intention and words of the buddhas and ancestors" are the everyday tea and rice of the buddhas and ancestors. The everyday fare of coarse tea and plain rice is "the intention and words of the buddhas and ancestors." The buddhas and ancestors make tea and rice; tea and rice maintain the buddhas and ancestors. (Dōgen, 2023: 291–292)

To succeed in the Buddhist tradition and transmit its truth is possible by following the example of the Buddhas and ancestors in their ordinary lives: eating rice and drinking tea. To put it in Christian terms, the truth transmitted through numerous Buddhas and ancestors is being incarnated in the non-extraordinary behaviors: eating rice and drinking tea.

4 Eating/Food Without Attachment and Discrimination

As mentioned earlier, the term "bodhisattva" in Mahayana Buddhism originally referred to Shakyamuni during his ascetic training in a previous life; however, the concept later expanded to encompass all ascetics. Among the legendary stories of Shakyamuni's previous lives, the most important is the story of his self-sacrifice. Another important story related to meat eating is the well-known story of the supreme sacrifice of King Śibi. Śibi, who was practicing almsgiving, saved a dove being chased by a hawk. However, the hawk pleaded with the king, saying that if it did not eat the dove's flesh, it would starve to death. The king granted the hawk's request and offered an equal quantity of his flesh to the hawk, saving both the dove and the hawk. But after all, the king had to offer all his flesh to the hawk because the hawk was so heavy (van Buitenen, 1975: 304).

In this story, which describes the extreme act of self-sacrifice for the sake of saving others, the king's body is given to the eagle, and both the eagle and the pigeon are saved, while the king himself dies. It is shown that in a situation where one cannot maintain one's own body without taking another's life and eating another's flesh, there is no choice but to do so. In such a situation, a Bodhisattva who would offer one's flesh to another would not accept eating another's flesh.

At the same time, the story of King Shibi teaches us about the boundary situation of human beings regarding eating/food. When we eat, we deprive another being of its life in whatever form, which also means that we have no other choice. In this sense, eating/food is "holy" in that it endows us with the energy of life, but eating/food teaches us that we are "humble" beings in that we deprive other beings of their lives for the sake of our own life (Ueki, 2016: 30).

And such an approach to eating/food finds itself as being intrinsically connected to the religious insight that "[r]eligions—especially biblical religions—introduce a clear distinction between need and desire by listing a series of precepts that regulate, though a balanced human relationship with food, an equally balanced human relationship with the world," in the sense that those relationships "involve transformative processes, which create new relationships," making us aware "the existence of other realities" (Fabris, 2024: vi, 68).

I believe that the Buddhist teaching of eating/food without attachment and the Christian understanding of eating/food without discrimination instruct us that the need must be addressed, and the desire should be controlled. When we realize, however, that addressing the need and controlling the desire are always broken along the way, the religious dimension of eating/food can be revealed in its true meaning. Non-attachment and non-discrimination describe not only the relationship between the eater and the eaten, but also the relationship between eaters in different cultures and religions.

As we have frequently experienced, interreligious dialogue often begins and ends with a verbal exchange of abstract, dogmatic self-assertions, where dialogue becomes a variation of ventriloquism. The issue of eating/food could be a soft catalyst for approaching interreligious dialogue in the realm of ordinary life. Above all, it will bring people from different religious traditions together, not in the conference room, but at the banquet table. Sitting together with people from different religious traditions and sharing the various "breads" of this world cooked in various ways, we hope to taste "the bread of the angels" (*lo pane de li angeli*) (Dante, *Convivio*) from above.

References

The bibliography on the topics covered is extensive. Therefore, below there is a list of both volumes and contributions cited in the text and authors, volumes, and contributions not cited but that are fundamental for the study and understanding of the topics referred to in this contribution.

Blofeld, J. (Trans.). (1962). *The Zen Teaching of Hui Hai on Sudden Illumination*. Rider & Company.

van Bragt, J. (2014). Christian Theology Learning from Buddhism. In J. W. Heisig & S. C. Kim (Eds.), *Interreligious Affinities: Encounters with the Kyoto School and the Religions of Japan* (pp. 43–53). Nanzan Institute for Religion and Culture.

Brillat-Savarin, J. A. (1970). *The Physiology of Taste* (A. Drayton, Trans.). Penguin Books.

van Buitenen, J. A. B. (Trans.). (1975). *The Mahābhārata* (Vol. 3). Chicago University Press.

Cha, J. S. (2008). Umsikgwa shiksaui sinhakjok jihyonghak: Shinyak songsorul jungsimuro [음식과 식사의 신학적 지형학: 신학성서를 중심으로 A Theological Topography of Food and Diet in the New Testament]. *Canon & Culture (A Journal of Biblical Interpretation in Context), 2*(2), 99–135.

Cleary, J. C. (Trans.). (1999). *Three Chan Classics*. Numata Center for Buddhist Translation and Research.

Dōgen. (1996a). *Instruction for the Tenzo* [典座教訓 *Tenzokyōkun*] (Daniel, L. T. Leighton & S. Okumura, Trans.). *Dōgen's Pure Standards for the Zen Community: A Translation of Eihei Shingi* (pp. 33–62). State University of New York Press.

Dōgen. (1996b). *The Dharma for Taking Food* [赴粥飯法 *Fushukuhanpō*] (Daniel, L. T. Leighton & S. Okumura, Trans.). *Dōgen's Pure Standards for the Zen Community: A Translation of Eihei Shingi* (pp. 83–108). State University of New York Press.

Dōgen. (2023). *Treasury of the True Dharma Eye* [正法眼蔵 *Dōgen's Shōbōgenzō*] (Vol. IV). The Administration Headquarters of Sōtō Zen Buddhism.

Douglas, M. (1971). Deciphering a Meal. In C Geertz (Ed.), *Myth, Symbol and Culture* (pp. 61–81). W. W. Norton & Company.

Fabris, A. (2024). *Ethics and Eating and Drinking: Food and Relations*. Springer Nature.

Furuyama, K. (2007). <*Fushukahanpō*>ni okeru <pōshishi, shishipō>ni zuite [『赴粥飯法』における「法是食・食是法」について A Study on Dōgen's Thought about Oneness of Meals and Dharma in *Fushukahanpō*]. *Journal of Sōtō Zen Studies, 49*, 1–6.

Henry, P. (Ed.). (2001). *Benedict's Dharma: Buddhists Reflect on the Rule of Saint Benedict*. New York.

Incandela, J. M. (1996). Playing God: Divine Activity, Human Activity, and Christian Ethics. *Cross Currents, 46*(1), 59–76.

Ingensiep, H. W., & Meinhardt, M. (2010). Introduction: Food Ethics in a Globalized World—Reality and Utopia. In F.-T. Gottwald, H. W. Ingensiep, & M. Meinhardt (Eds.), *Food Ethics* (pp. 1–14). Springer.

Jenks, A. W. (1992). Eating and Drinking in the Old Testament. In D. N. Freedman (Ed.), *Anchor Bible Dictionary* (Vol. 2, pp. 250–254). Doubleday.

Kim, S. C. (2008). *Kami to idenshi: Idenkōgaku jidai niokeru kirisutokyō* [神と遺伝子:遺伝子工学時代におけるキリスト教] *God and Gene: Christianity in the age of Genetic Engineering*. Kyōbunkan.

Kim, S. C. (2016). Religion and Science in Dialogue: An Asian Christian View. *Zygon: Journal of Religion and Science, 51*(1), 63–70.

Kim, S. C. (2022). *The Center is Everywhere: Christianity in Dialogue with Religion and Science*. Pickwick Publications.

Koga, H. (1991). *Dictionary for Zen Words*. Shibunkaku Publishing.

Mepham, B. (1996). Ethical Analysis of Food Biotechnologies: An Evaluative Framework. In B. Mepham (Ed.), *Food Ethics* (pp. 101–119). Routledge.

Nam, C. (2021). Jonggyosha yonguui choigun gyonghyan: Umshik yongusarul jungsimuro [종교사 연구의 최근 경향: 음식 연구사를 중심으로 The Recent Trends in the Study of Religious History: Especially Focusing on the Historiography of Food History]. *Humanities Studies East and West, 60*, 213–247.

Poceski, M. (2006). *Guishan jingce* (*Guishan's Admonitions*) and the Ethical Foundations of Chan Practice. In S. Heine & D. S. Wright (Eds.), *Zen Classics. Formative Texts in the History of Zen Buddhism* (pp. 15–42). Oxford University Press.

Poceski, M. (2007). *Ordinary Mind as the Way: The Hongzhou School and the Growth of Chan Buddhism*. Oxford University Press.

Shohei, I. (Trans.). (2006). *The Baizhang Zen Monastic Regulations*. Numata Center for Buddhist Translations and Research.

Sister Vajira, & Story, F. (Transl.). (1964). *Last Days of the Buddha. The Mahāparinibbāna Sutta*. Buddhist Publication Society.

Sloterdijk, P. (1999). *Regeln für den Menschenpark: Ein Antwortschreiben zu Heideggers Brief über den Humanismus*. Suhrkamp.
Tarocco, F., Rossi, A., Zhang, B. W., & Francescon, S. (2024). Eating Like a Buddhist: Vegetarianism and Ethical Foodscapes in the Twenty-First Century. *Annali di Ca'Foscari. Serie orientale, 60*, 257–286.
Ueki, K. (2016). Taberukotowa singakuno kadaito naruka: taberukoto karano toito karadano henyō" [食べることは神学の課題となるか:食べることからの問いと身体の変容 Is Eating a Theological Agenda?: Question Through Eating and Transformation of Body]. *The Bulletin of Institute for Christian Studies Meiji Gakuin University, 48*, 25–53.
Yorizumi, M. (2009). Bukkyō niokeru shoku" [仏教における「食」 A study of Dietary Thought in Buddhism]. *The 3rd Consortium on Global Perspectives in Japanese Studies,* 301–309.

Law

The Concept of Integral Wellbeing in the International and National Regulatory Framework

Francesco Bruno and Ginevra Brutto

1 Introduction: The Notion of Wellbeing

> The States parties to this Constitution declare, in conformity with the Charter of the United Nations, that the following principles are basic to the happiness, harmonious relations and security of all peoples: Health is a state of complete physical, mental and social wellbeing and not merely the absence of disease or infirmity.[1] The enjoyment of the highest attainable standard of health is one of the fundamental rights of every human being without distinction of race, religion, political belief, economic or

[1] This article is part of the outputs of the project "*Integral WELLbeing for human flourishing: healthcare and food from an ethical and legal perspective (I-WELL)*" funded by the European Union under the National Recovery and Resilience Plan (PNRR), Mission 4, Component 2, Investment 1.1 "Fund for the National Research Program and Projects of Significant National Interest (PRIN)" (Prot. no. P2022MFWB9, Sector ERC SH2, CUP C53D23009930001).

F. Bruno (✉) · G. Brutto
Campus Bio-Medico University of Rome, Rome, Italy
e-mail: francesco.bruno@unicampus.it

F. Bruno et al. (eds.), *Healthcare and Food*,
https://doi.org/10.1007/978-981-95-5899-5_8

> social condition. The health of all people is fundamental to the attainment of peace and security and is dependent upon the fullest co-operation of individuals and States. The achievement of any State in the promotion and protection of health is of value to all (Constitution of The World Health Organization—WHO).[2]

The preamble to the WHO Constitution represents, still today, the most important legal reference in the debate on the concept of wellbeing. The definition provided by the WHO focuses on the logical contrast between health and the absence of disease or infirmity. In this context, health is a psycho-physical state in which "social wellbeing" represents the third element of the whole required to achieve happiness, harmonious relations, and security of all people. However, the process of defining the concept becomes complicated when we realize that the notion of

> wellbeing constitutes a multifaceted concept that presents several connotations and can be analyzed from different perspectives. The term can be defined in many ways depending on the context in which it is considered; for instance, the "wellbeing of a person" can be identified with what is intrinsically valuable in relation to someone and what is good for that person, while "subjective wellbeing" refers to individuals' personal sense of how well their lives are going (Boday et al., 2024).

Over time, there have been various attempts to define the concept in the fields of medicine, anthropology, and social sciences, which have had definite influence in the legal field. There are three main theories that have been used to identify the specific elements of wellbeing to classify its

---

G. Brutto
e-mail: g.brutto@unicampus.it

[2] The Constitution was adopted by the International Health Conference held in New York from 19 June to 22 July 1946, signed on 22 July 1946 by the representatives of 61 States (Off. Rec. Wld Hlth Org., 2, 100) and entered into force on 7 April 1948. Amendments adopted by the Twenty-sixth, Twenty-ninth, Thirty-ninth, and Fifty-first World Health Assemblies (resolutions WHA26.37, WHA29.38, WHA39.6 and WHA51.23) came into force on 3 February 1977, 20 January 1984, 11 July 1994 and 15 September 2005 respectively and are incorporated in the present text.

perception: the hedonic theory (Moore, 2019), the desire theory (Heathwood, 2019), and the objective list theory (Fletcher, 2013; Lin, 2014). The historical and growing interest in the concept

> dates back thousands of years, with complex indigenous understandings through to the ancient Greeks. The notion of wellbeing has endured the test of time and is contemporarily central to the social sciences. As Alexandrova highlights, "concern with human wellbeing is at the very root of modern social science thus began its life as a form of knowledge devoted officially to the advancement of wellbeing". Particularly interesting, however, is that 'wellbeing' also constitutes an emergent hot topic across the social sciences, with disciplines ranging from psychology and economics to sociology, philosophy, literature, developmental studies, health, communication and media, education, public policy and beyond, all placing greater emphasis on the term and construct than previously. It is clear that the rapid and phenomenal growth of the field of positive psychology has contributed to stimulating interest in wellbeing more broadly. Today, many scholars across most social science discipline, at least from a publishing perspective, are taking a wellbeing-oriented lens to their field and discipline. Additionally, beyond academia and in the realm of popular culture (at least in western societies), wellbeing is becoming more central in various dialogues, with the acknowledgment that wellbeing (in contrast to illbeing) is important for everyone. For example, Seligman notes that when parents are asked what they most want for their children, wellbeing is usually present in their answers and also usually at the top of the list (Jarden & Roache, 2023).

Starting from the multidisciplinary interest that the concept of wellbeing has raised, the research will attempt to reconstruct the applicable international and European regulatory framework and the legal conditions which allow people to achieve integral wellbeing, both individual and collective, from a food health point of view. The work focused on the analysis of said current normative instruments striving to develop a legal foundation of the integral wellbeing guided by food and nutrition, as a driver of change to promote a more sustainable future.

2 The International Level

Given its multidisciplinary relevance, the analysis covered in this paper aims to define the relevance of the concept of wellbeing within the legal framework. For this reason, it is necessary to begin the analysis at the international law level.

In the field of law, wellbeing is usually approached through the protection of a "constellation" of rights—health, social security, education, housing, work, a healthy environment, privacy, and family life—paired with state duties to respect, protect, and fulfill these rights. In modern times, the first recognition of the relevance of the concept of wellbeing can be traced back to the signing of the WHO Constitution in 1946. «Participants of this solidary Conference, assembled within a year of the end of the Second World War, apparently got along so well with each other that virtually no disagreement on the essentials occurred» (Ip, 2020) hence the delegates felt a strong urge to embody the global sentiment that public health should be given extraordinarily high priority in the nascent UN system (Lee, 2009). The WHO Constitution was in some sense 'more ambitious than the UN Charter in terms of its goals' (Alvarez, 2017). The Constitution's expressive Preamble confidently redefines the concept of health as «a state of complete physical, mental, and social wellbeing and not merely the absence of disease or infirmity», which is «one of the fundamental rights of every human being without distinction of race, religion, political belief, economic or social condition». It proceeds to declare that «The health of all people» is «fundamental to the attainment of peace and security», and is «dependent upon the fullest co-operation of individuals»; and so to condemn «[u]nequal development in different countries in the promotion of health and control of disease, especially communicable disease» to be «a common danger». It moreover avers, «healthy development of the child» is of «basic importance»; and the dissemination of «medical, psychological and related knowledge» is «essential to the fullest attainment of health» (Ip, 2020).[3]

[3] For an analysis of the normativity of the WHO Constitution, please refer to the article by Ip, E.C. (2020) which analyzes «how the discordance between the WHO's official purposes and its

In 1948 wellbeing is once again mentioned in the Universal Declaration of Human Rights (UDHR). After defining the concepts of freedom and equality (Articles 1 and 2), individual rights (Articles 3 to 11), the rights of individuals in relation to the community (Articles 12 to 17) and fundamental freedoms (freedom of thought, opinion, religion and conscience, freedom of expression and peaceful association in Articles 18 to 21), Articles 22 to 27 of the UDHR define economic, social and cultural rights. These include the first explicit recognition of personal wellbeing as an essential part of the right to freedom from poverty, since:

> everyone has the right to a standard of living adequate for the health and wellbeing of himself and of his family, including food, clothing, housing and medical care and necessary social services, and the right to security in the event of unemployment, sickness, disability, widowhood, old age or other lack of livelihood in circumstances beyond his control (Art. 25.1 UDHR).

The real novelty introduced by the UDHR was that for the first time in international law, individuals were no longer only considered as members of a group (the states) or a minority/category of the group. They became the object of protection as individuals.

Innovative in theory, this "proclamation without enforceable protection" (i.e. the UDHR (Cassese, 2005)) inspired other more effective instruments of international law including the International Covenant on Economic, Social and Cultural Rights (known as the ICESCR), signed twenty years after the adoption of the UDHR. The ICESCR, adopted in 1966 and entered into force in 1976, affirms the right to the highest attainable standard of physical and mental health, adequate food, housing, social security, education, and conditions of work. It requires progressive realization using maximum available resources, prohibits discrimination, and recognizes minimum core obligations (e.g., essential primary health care) that must be met even in resource-constrained settings. The International Covenant on Civil and Political

---

constitutional competencies has played out since its inception. It identifies five major constitutional constraints that have effectively barred the Organization from asserting its legislative authority to produce a corpus of 'hard' international treaty law on public health».

Rights (ICCPR) complements the framework provided by ICESCR by protecting life, body integrity, privacy, and family life rights that function as enabling conditions for wellbeing by imposing both negative duties (do not interfere) and positive obligations (take reasonable steps to safeguard).

Other specialized international law instruments have also referred to the obligations of States to respect, protect, and fulfill wellbeing: the Convention on the Rights of the Child (CRC) secures children's rights to health, development, social protection and education; the Convention on the Rights of Persons with Disabilities (CRPD) reframes disability through accessibility, inclusion, independent living and community support. Lastly, the International Labour Organization (ILO) corpus establishes that decent work conditions are pillars of wellbeing, from occupational safety and health to social security and fair remuneration.

At the regional level, there is no explicit recognition of the concept of wellbeing, but rights such as health, social security, and education are recognized. The American Convention on Human Rights and the Protocol of San Salvador protect health, social security, and education. The Inter-American Court has pioneered expansive readings of the right to life and dignity to cover environmental harms, access to water, and protection of vulnerable communities, making wellbeing a justiciable concern. It is interesting to note how the experience of the African continent stands out for its references to the wellbeing of communities. Given the fact that the African Charter on Human and Peoples' Rights recognizes both the right to health and the right to a general satisfactory environment favorable to development, the African Commission on Human and Peoples' Rights (ACHPR Commission) and the African Court on Human and Peoples' Rights (ACHRP Court) have linked community wellbeing to land, culture, participation, and freedom from environmental degradation. There are rulings three[4] that address

[4] The case of Endorois v. Kenya, ACHPR Comm. 276/2003, criticizes Kenya for failing to ensure the continued improvement of the Endorois' wellbeing after their removal from ancestral lands. The ACHPR Commission treats Endorois' community wellbeing as the yardstick of the right to development, linking it to secure land, cultural and religious life, access to resources/benefit-sharing, and effective participation. In the "Ogoni case" (Serac & Cesr v. Nigeria, ACHPR Comm. 155/96), massive pollution and destruction of farmlands and fisheries were connected to health, subsistence/livelihood, and a satisfactory environment as components of

the concept of wellbeing essentially linking it to loss of ancestral territory, environmental and health protection.

More recently, wellbeing, as a concept connected to health, freedom from poverty and environmental protection, has found its way into international law instruments that, since the late 1990s,[5] aim to regulate measures to combat climate change and promote sustainable ecological transition.

Sustainable development was first defined in the Brundtland Report as "development that meets the needs of the present without compromising the ability of future generations to meet their own needs." It has been the subject of three world conferences on the environment and the resolution adopted in September 2015 by the United Nations General Assembly *Transforming our world: the 2030 Agenda for Sustainable Development*, and the basis for the latest international positions on biodiversity and climate change. Today, the "sustainable development of the Earth" is an integral part of the European Union's overall objectives. The international community's latest major commitment to sustainable development was expressed with the 2030 Agenda which approved the 17 Sustainable Development goals (hereafter "SDGs"). The Agenda now recognizes its importance calling on states to «ensure healthy lives and promote wellbeing for all at all ages» hence

> sustainable development must be achieved in its three dimensions – economic, social and environmental – in a balanced and integrated manner. The 2030 Agenda is aimed at all states in the world, not only

---

collective wellbeing of the communities impacted. Lastly the ACHRP Court in the Ogiek v. Kenya case (App. No. 006/2012) finds violations of collective property, culture/religion, natural resources, development, and non-discrimination, recognizing that eviction from Mau Forest undermined the Ogiek's cultural survival, livelihoods, and decision-making power-key pillars of wellbeing.

[5] Sustainable development was first defined in the Brundtland Report as «development that meets the needs of the present without compromising the ability of future generations to meet their own needs». It has been the subject of three world conferences on the environment (the Rio summit in 1992, the Johannesburg summit in 2002, and the Rio+20 summit, also held in Rio, in 2012) and the resolution adopted in September 2015 by the United Nations General Assembly "Transforming our world: the 2030 Agenda for Sustainable Development," and the basis for the latest international positions on biodiversity and climate change. Today, the "sustainable development of the Earth" is an integral part of the European Union's overall objectives.

> because of the obvious involvement of the richest countries in achieving the SDGs on environmental sustainability, but also because of the focus on economic and, above all, social sustainability. Even though there are developed countries ruled by law, with democratic governments, there are people who lack from wellbeing (food, health, education, equality…), mainly linked to situations of poverty, whose rates have suffered important declinations due to the Covid-19 pandemic in almost every country (Martinón Quintero, 2023).

In this context, the social aspect of sustainable development refers to ensuring people's wellbeing in relation to economic development and environmental protection and focuses primarily on poverty and exclusion.

> From a human rights perspective, social sustainability as the social dimension of sustainable development involves talking about the physical, emotional and social needs of human beings. It «emphasizes living in ways that can be sustained because they are healthy and satisfying for people and communities. This requires providing for material, social and emotional needs, avoiding behaviors that result in poor health, emotional distress and conflict»; it is identified with the wellbeing which includes food, housing, clean water, health, education, and personal security. In this sense, it implies a questioning of the mere economic growth as the privileged option for progress, going beyond GDP to pay attention to objective and subjective components of wellbeing: «Sustainable human development adds a social dimension to this already difficult balance between economic development and respect for the environment: social inclusion and the fight against poverty. In classical economics, GDP growth was compatible with exclusion and socio-economic inequalities. Distribution did not matter. On the contrary, the human dimension of development takes up this challenge to achieve social inclusion, equal opportunities and real equality between men and women» (Martinón Quintero, 2023).

3 The Role of Wellbeing in European Legislation

> The Union's aim is to promote peace, its values and the wellbeing of its peoples (Article 3 of Treaty on European Union – TEU).

In EU law, wellbeing is not a single justiciable right but a constitutional objective (TEU), a binding obligation for health and social concerns (Treaty on the functioning of European Union—TFEU), and a policy lens used to craft and evaluate legislation. According to this perspective, the legislative history of the European Union records a series of regulatory areas, such as health and safety at workplace discipline and animal welfare within food law, in which the concept of wellbeing represents one of the fundamental components to be pursued and a tool for assessing regulatory compliance itself.

> Regarding the wellbeing of workers, it can be said that the notion is closely linked to the definition of health as formulated by the Constitution of the World Health Organization (WHO) in 1946 ... Nonetheless, this definition has been criticized on two fronts: first and foremost, due to the utopian nature of the definition, which evokes an idealized state that is unattainable for any individual on account of the use of the term "complete". In fact, by classifying all people as unhealthy, it implies that everyone is eligible for corrective medical intervention, an approach that may not correspond to the reality of different health conditions. A second criticism is directed at the lack of an explicit reference to the concept of wellbeing in the WHO definition: "flourishing" – which can be seen as a synonymous of "the power to be" or "the ability to adapt and self-manage" – is important in the contemporary interpretation of health. Understanding these issues is critical in order to correctly frame the debate regarding employees' wellbeing, as it recognizes the complexities and nuances involved in the definition and promotion of health in different occupational contexts (Boday et al., 2024).

Improving health and safety at work has been an important concern for the EU since the 1980s. Legislation at European level sets minimum standards for the protection of workers, while allowing Member States maintaining or introduce more stringent measures. Health and safety at work is a key component of the European Pillar of Social Rights Action Plan. Based on Article 153 TFEU, the EU can adopt legislation on health and safety at work to support and complement the activities of the Member States.

> In Europe, the awareness of the need for a system regulating occupational health and safety emerged during the 19th-century Industrial Revolution: the shift of a large workforce from rural areas to urban centers for employment in burgeoning industries prompted workers to organize to protect and defend their health and safety at the workplace and their own wellbeing, which increasingly became widespread and gained prominence as an issue, leading to the enactment of legal provisions. In this early developmental phase, legislation gradually recognized the importance to ensure more humane working conditions. This development led to increase the understanding of how much influence has the workplace on worker health, as well as on worker wellbeing, which again affects the productivity and the good ongoing of the company (Boday et al., 2024).

Under the auspices of the European Coal and Steel Community, various research programs were carried out in the field. The need for a global approach to the matter became manifest with the establishment of the European Economic Community (EEC) in 1957. The Advisory Committee on Safety, Hygiene and Health Protection at Work was set up in 1974 to assist the Commission. Achieving minimum levels of protection was necessary to complete the EU single market, so a number of directives were adopted, including metallic lead, asbestos, and noise. The adoption of the Single European Act in 1987 brought health and safety at work into the EEC Treaty for the first time, in an article laying down minimum requirements and allowing the Council to adopt occupational health and safety directives by qualified majority. The aims were: to improve workers' health and safety at work; to harmonise conditions in the working environment; to prevent 'social dumping'; and to prevent companies from moving to areas with a lower level of protection in order to gain a competitive edge.

In this context, it is important to emphasize that, from the outset, European legislators recognized wellbeing as one of the fundamental components of workers' rights. The link was immediately made and still is with the productivity of economic systems, which would be improved by the possibility for workers to operate in a healthy, safe, and hazard-free environment. In recent years, especially after the SARS-CoV-2 pandemic, during which the global labor market was forced to adapt by implementing new and more pervasive remote working mechanisms, the concept of wellbeing at work has expanded to encompass the issues of smart and remote working.

> In a broader sense, the protection of workers' wellbeing in the workplace and work-life balance become decisive parameters to select a job when demand of employees is high ... [In this context] the concept of part-time work is often seen as a type of employment relationship that is not immediately associated with improving worker conditions. After all, it is frequently considered more as a flexibility element in the employment contract beneficial to the employer, who can determine the work period most suitable for their business structure regardless of the worker's needs. However, this perspective is shortsighted and fails to consider the potential of this institution and the regulatory framework governing it. For instance, the Council Directive 97/81/EC of 15 December 1997 concerning the Framework Agreement on part-time work can be analysed, especially regarding the part in which it states «(3) Whereas point 7 of the Community Charter of the Fundamental Social Rights of Workers provides, inter alia, that 'the completion of the internal market must lead to an improvement in the living and working conditions of workers in the European Community. This process must result from an approximation of these conditions while the improvement is being maintained, as regards in particular (...) forms of employment other than open-ended contracts, such as fixed-term contracts, parttime working, temporary work, and seasonal work'». In this perspective, part-time work, is considered a tool to enhance working conditions for workers rather than a flexibility tool for employers or a specific risk factor. It is crucial to acknowledge within the concept of health protection the definition of the WHO Constitution and the specific interpretation of the CJUE, which "broadens the

> concept of risk from mere physical to psychical and psychosocial, thus emphasising the relevance of the workplace as 'environment' where the worker has the right to each a state of complete physical, mental, and social wellbeing" (Boday et al., 2024).

Leaving for now aside the role of wellbeing in European food law (topic that will be covered in the next paragraph), the principle imposed by Article 3 of the TEU led to the inclusion of the concept of wellbeing in the European Union's economic planning, leading to the creation of the theory known as "Economy of Wellbeing."

This topic of great interest in the international socio-economic debate was the subject of a conclusion adopted by the Council of the European Union on October 24, 2019, on the economy of wellbeing. Based on the work carried out by the Organisation for Economic Co-operation and Development (OECD),[6] the Council calls on the European Commission and Member States to integrate a cross-sectoral perspective of the economy of wellbeing into all EU and Member State policy areas stating that:

> people's wellbeing is a principal aim of the European Union. The Economy of Wellbeing brings into focus the raison d'être of the Union as enshrined in the Treaties and in the Charter of Fundamental Rights of the European Union. The creation of an environment that enables people to reach their full potential and to enjoy their fundamental rights is a central component of the Economy of Wellbeing. At the same time, sustainable and inclusive economic growth and resilience function as enablers for the wellbeing of people, societies and the planet. … The balance between economic growth and social progress lies at the heart of European integration. … The Organisation for Economic Cooperation and Development has emphasized that investing in improved health, education, employment, gender equality and social protection for all members of society contributes to economic growth. In addition,

[6] The forerunner of the OECD was the Organisation for European Economic Co-operation (OEEC), which was formed to administer American and Canadian aid under the Marshall Plan for the reconstruction of Europe after World War II. The Convention transforming the OEEC into the OECD was signed at the Chateau de la Muette in Paris on December 14, 1960, and entered into force on 30 September 1961.

> the social returns associated with greater individual wellbeing—including greater trust, more civic engagement and social cohesion—contribute to economic growth through stronger total factor productivity, greater financial and political stability, and enhanced resilience to adverse shocks. The Economy of Wellbeing is also at the heart of the United Nations 2030 Agenda for Sustainable Development to which all Member States are committed. Along the same lines, the importance of investing in health, social protection and education has been recognized by several international organizations, namely the World Bank Group, the International Monetary Fund, the International Labour Organization and the World Health Organization (The Economy of Wellbeing Council Conclusions, 2019/C 400/09).

The OECD document and the Council decision represent an interesting "formalization" of a legislative trend that is well established in the recent history of the European Union. The topic, which has clearly been affected by events related first to the SARS-CoV-2 pandemic and then to the invasion of Ukrainian territory, does not appear to have been followed up in other formal documents, but its objectives are consistent with the regulatory framework on food law and One Health since the Council explicitly calls the Member States and the European Commission to:

> DEVELOP a cross-sectoral assessment of impacts on wellbeing in order to strengthen knowledge-based policy and decision-making.
> CONSIDER using indicators related to wellbeing to monitor and report national budget processes and for knowledge-based decision-making. All these indicators should be disaggregated by sex. …
> INCLUDE an Economy of Wellbeing perspective horizontally into national and Union policies and put people and their wellbeing at the centre of policy design.
> IMPLEMENT evidence-based and effective policy interventions at national and Union level to address common challenges to wellbeing.
> …
> CONTINUE to develop rigorous quantitative and qualitative data collection and statistical methods for measuring and regularly monitoring

people's wellbeing in order to provide, together with the economic indicators in the context of the European Semester, a comprehensive analysis as a basis for policy and decision-making.

4 The Concept of Wellbeing in European Food Law: From Animal Welfare to the One Health Approach

Although food undoubtedly represents a fundamental part of the concept of health and food law pursues the ambitious goal of combining the principles of food safety, food health, and food security[7] with the pursuit of the right to health, it is interesting to note that the word "wellbeing" is almost virtually never used in food law legislative vocabulary. While the concept, in its complex and multidisciplinary dimension that we have come to know, is clearly present in many aspects, historically explicit reference to wellbeing can be found in animal welfare legislation.

While it is true that the protection of animals during slaughter has been regulated at European level since Directive 1974/577/EEC, transposed in Italy by Law No. 439 of August 2, 1978, followed by Directive 1993/119/EC, also relating to the protection of animals during slaughter or killing, implemented in Italy by Legislative Decree No. 333 of September 1, 1998, replaced by Regulation 1099/2009 of September 24, 2009, adopted using Article 37 as its legal basis, it is clear that it was in the last years of the 20th century that a genuine Community law on animals began to emerge and take shape, especially after the BSE syndrome

---

[7] Based on internationally accepted definitions, formalized by EU law, food safety refers to "the health and hygiene safety of food products in terms of health protection, taken in the broadest sense throughout the entire food chain and including consumer communication tools," and food security refers to "the economic and physical security of having sufficient food available to meet normal dietary needs." The most recent formulations of food safety and food security "have added complexity to these definitions, bringing essential elements of food safety back into food security, because there can be no security of supply if it is not hygienically safe, and placing within food safety a whole series of elements of quality and compliance with standards that go beyond the simple minimum guarantee of hygiene."

> prompted the adoption of a series of innovative and reactive regulations (Saija, 2024).

Although the use of the word "welfare" may suggest an intention to care for animals consumed as food, in reality the inclusion of ethical issues in animal legislation is more recent than the historical intentions that started European legislation on the subject. Actually:

> doctrine has not failed to highlight how the interventions prepared by the European legislator even before the adoption of the Maastricht Treaty of 1992, the establishment of the European Union, and the Amsterdam Treaty of 1997 (amending the Treaty on the European Community, including Protocol 33, which identifies animal welfare as an autonomous objective of guarantee and protection in the light of human-centered logic)—documents which marked the turning point in the European perspective of animal welfare as a biocentric science—were nothing more than an expression of the mediated character entrusted to the protection of animals and aimed at satisfying them; principally, for further and different purposes: the protection of human health, the completion of the Single European Market, the functioning of the Common Agricultural Policy, the safeguarding of consumer interests and beliefs, environmental protection, etc (Pisciotta Tosini, 2025).

This mediated "function" of animal welfare legislation can be further observed if we consider how:

> in recent years we have witnessed a shift in the anthropocentric perspective on which the animal welfare debate was based in the past. On the other hand, when discussing the protection of animals during slaughter, we cannot ignore the European Commission's continued stance on the matter, namely that the high standards required in terms of animal welfare are not only and exclusively functional to improving the health of animals, but also to ensuring a better quality of the food obtained from them, without neglecting economic considerations, such as the reduction in the need for drugs with a consequent favorable impact on biodiversity. Together with sustainability, this is one of the fundamental keys to understanding the current European food system, and with this in mind,

> legislators are also taking steps to achieve a series of objectives that are compatible with these principles (Saija, 2024).

This trend therefore links the concept of animal welfare primarily to the achievement of food safety, food health, and food security objectives, and only secondarily to ethical issues directly related to the consideration of animals as "sentient beings" and, more often, to issues of religious rights protection.

Beyond the historical centrality of animal welfare, the contemporary European food law progressively embeds a broader One Health perspective, i.e., the integrated governance of risks and opportunities at the human, animal, and environment interface.

> The term One Health was introduced at the beginning of the new millennium and highlights the growing awareness of how global health requires a multisectoral approach capable of integrating the analysis of environmental, chemical-physical, and biological parameters (plants, microorganisms, animals). In particular, this term recognizes the interdependence of human health with that of domestic and wild animals, plants, and the entire ecosystem (De Gara et al. 2022).

One Health translates into regulatory techniques that coordinate food safety and nutrition policies with animal health, plant health, and environmental protection, thus using the concept of wellbeing as a cross-cutting objective rather than a sectoral aspiration. In EU law this integration is visible both at constitutional level where wellbeing is framed as a Union aim (i.e., Article 3 TEU) and across ordinary legislation shaping reforms for the food systems, official controls, and market operators' responsibilities.

This trend can be seen in recent reforms to general food law (i.e., Regulation No 178/2002) and the system of risk analysis that gradually evolved toward integrated assessments by European Food Safety Authority (EFSA) in collaboration with European Centre for Disease Prevention and Control (ECDC) and environmental authorities, so that hazard identification and exposure assessment account for zoonotic dynamics, antimicrobial resistance (AMR), chemical contaminants and ecological stressors along the food chain. This approach is reinforced by: (i) the Official Controls Regulation (i.e., Regulation No 2017/625), which unifies control modalities across food and feed, animal health and welfare, plant health and plant protection products, facilitating horizontal enforcement and data sharing and (ii) the European Farm to Fork strategy has given a systemic policy home to One Health within the European Green Deal, coupling food safety with nutrition quality, sustainability targets, and resilience of supply chains.

In this context, it is important to emphasize that the One Health approach strengthens the connection link between individual and population wellbeing with ecosystem integrity, aligning market freedoms with non-market constitutional objectives (health, high level of consumer protection, environmental protection), and consolidating the legal foundations for integral wellbeing in the agri-food domain.

5 Conclusions

International and European law do not confine "wellbeing" into a single, justiciable right; nevertheless, in the agri-food sector, the trajectory from food safety to food system sustainability—via animal welfare and now One Health—shows how wellbeing functions as a unifying legal rationale connecting individual entitlements (health, right to food and sustainable food) with collective goods (public health, ecosystem resilience, social cohesion).

From this reconstruction, at least four normative implications emerge. First, wellbeing requires preventive and integrated risk governance: precaution, surveillance, and source-control are not optional add-ons but structural requirements where scientific uncertainty and interdependence prevail. Second, the right to food must be read in its contemporary, three-dimensional form—food safety, food health, and food security—so that regulatory choices promote healthy diets and equitable access while respecting planetary boundaries. Third, animal welfare is both a value in itself and a means to human and environmental wellbeing. Fourth, policy evaluation should incorporate wellbeing indicators alongside economic metrics, in line with the Union's economy-of-wellbeing perspective, to better capture the social returns of health-promoting food policies going beyond GPD.

In conclusion, One Health provides the legal grammar for "integral wellbeing" in European food law: it justifies horizontal coordination, data coordination, and preventive regulation; it bridges ethics and efficiency in animal welfare; and it translates the Union's constitutional aim of promoting the wellbeing of its peoples into concrete, justiciable standards across the food chain. Through these avenues, the legal system can make food and nutrition a driver of change toward a healthier, more resilient, and inclusive future for individuals and communities.[8]

References

Adler, A., & Seligman, M. E. P. (2016). Using wellbeing for public policy: Theory, measurement, and recommendations. *In International Journal of Wellbeing, 6*(1), 1–35. https://doi.org/10.5502/ijw.v6i1.429

Adornato, F., Albisinni, F., & Germanò, A. (2010). *Agricoltura e Alimentazione–Principi e regole della qualità: disciplina internazionale, comunitaria, nazionale*. Giuffré.

Albisinni, F. (2015). Le declinazioni della sicurezza alimentare. In Albisinni, F. *Strumentario di diritto alimentare europeo*. 5th Edition. Utet.

Albisinni, F., & Costato, L. (2023). *Trattato breve di diritto agrario e dell'Unione Europea*. IV Edition. Wolters Kluver.

Alexandrova, A. (2017). *A philosophy for the science of well-being*. Oxford University Press.

Alvarez, J.E. (2017). *The Impact of International Organizations on International Law*. Brill.

Angner, E. (2011). The evolution of eupathics: The historical roots of subjective measures of well-being. *International Journal of Wellbeing, 1*(1), 4–41.

Benozzo, M. (2023). *Biotecnologie agroalimentari e nuove tecniche di miglioramento genetico tra Unione Europea e Stati Uniti*. Aracne.

[8] The bibliography on the topics covered is extensive. Therefore, below there is a list of both volumes and contributions cited in the text and authors, volumes, and contributions that are fundamental for the study and understanding of the topics referred to in this contribution.

Bengoetxea, J. (2020). Introducción. In Consejo vasco del movimiento europeo, Eurobasque (Ed.), *Sostenibilidad de la Europa del s. XXI: económica, ambiental y social*. Eurobasque.
Boday, N. S., Campensan, D., Pavin, A., & Valenti, C. (2024). The concept of "well-being" in (and outside) the workplace. *Diritto della sicurezza sul Lavoro*, 1/2024.
Bolognini, S. (2013). Food safety e comunicazione ai cittadini in materia di sicurezza e di rischio alimentari: il concetto di prodotto alimentare insicuro al vaglio della Corte di giustizia. In *Riv. dir. agr.*
Bolognini, S. (2022). PAC, sostenibilità e bioeconomia. In S. Masini & V. Rubino (Eds.), *La sostenibilità in agricoltura e la riforma della PAC*. Cacucci.
Borghi, P. (2003). Sicurezza alimentare e commercio internazionale. In Rook Basile, E., Massart, A., Germanò, A. (Eds.), *Prodotti agricoli e sicurezza alimentare—Atti del VII Congresso mondiale di Diritto agrario dell'Unione Mondiale degli Agraristi Universitari in memoria di Louis Lorvellec*, volume I.
Bruno, F. (2000a). Il principio di precauzione tra diritto dell'Unione Europea e WTO. In *Dir. e giur. agr. e ambiente*.
Bruno, F. (2000b). Principio di precauzione e organismi geneticamente modificati. In *Dir. e giur. agr. e ambiente* (II/2000).
Bruno, F. (2017). Il diritto alimentare nel contesto globale: USA e UE a confronto. Cedam.
Bruno, F. (2022). Il diritto alimentare. Sviluppo sostenibile e tutela della salute. Cedam.
Brutto, G. (2025). Diritto al cibo e diritto ad un cibo sostenibile. In *Teoria*, 2025/2 n. 46.
Cafaro, P. (2015). Sicurezza e benessere economico. In *Rivista di polizia* (1–2/2015).
Canfora, I. (2018). Le imprese alimentari e la protezione del benessere animale nelle società multiculturali. In *Agricoltura Istituzioni Mercati*, 1/2018.
Cassese, A. (2015). *I diritti umani oggi*. Gius. Laterza & Figli Spa.
Carmignani, S. (2024). Acqua e agricoltura: una prospettiva di economia circolare. In *Studi Senesi*.
Costato, L. (2011). Dalla food security alla food insecurity. In *Rivista di diritto agrario* (1/2011).
Costato, L. (2017). Diritto al cibo e Global Food Security: la perdurante assenza di un'adeguata risposta europea. In *Rivista di diritto alimentare* (4/2017).
Costato, L. (2018). Il ritorno alla Food Security. In *Rivista di diritto alimentare* (1/2008).

Costello, J. (2019). *Workplace wellbeing—A relational approach*. Routledge.
Crisp, R. (2021). Well-Being. In *The Stanford Encyclopaedia of Philosophy*, Metaphysics Research Lab of the Stanford University.
De Gara, L., Gherardi, M. (2022). Modelli di analisi con metodologie innovative del rischio di esposizione ad agenti chimici e biologici in agricoltura in ottica "one health". In *Rivista degli infortuni e delle malattie professionali* (2/ 2022).
Di Lauro, A. (2024). Innovazione nel mercato agroalimentare fra "rotture simboliche" e "norme tecniche". In *Sfide del diritto agrario nell'epoca attuale, XVI Congresso Mondiale di diritto agrario e V Congresso Mondiale di Diritto amazzonico.*
Dornisch, S. (2022). The Evolution of Well-Being: An Anthropology-Based, Multidisciplinary Review. In *Humans*. doi:https://doi.org/10.3390/humans 2040011.
Eger, R.J., Maridal, J.H. (2015). A statistical meta-analysis of the wellbeing literature. In *Int. J. Wellbeing*.
Fletcher, G. (2013). A Fresh Start for an Objective List Theory of Well-Being. in *Utilitas*.
Fracchia, F. (2010). 2. The "formation" of the concept: from the Brundtland Report to the so-called environmental code, according to the principles-rules-principles sequence. Chapter I in (Same author) *Sustainable Development: The Weak Voice of the Other between Environmental Protection and the Protection of the Human Species.*
Gatchel, R. J., & Kishino, N. D. (2012). Conceptual approaches to occupational health and wellness: An overview. In R. J. Gatchel & I. Z. Schultz (Eds.), *Handbook of occupational health and wellness*. Springer.
Giubboni, S., & Rossi, A. (2012). *Infortuni sul lavoro e risarcimento del danno.* Giuffrè.
Germanò, A. (2022). Manuale di diritto agrario. IX edition. G. Giappichelli.
Hammer, L. B., & Brady, J. M. (2020). The evolution of worker well-being and work-life issues. In L. Koppes Bryan (Ed.), *Historical perspectives in industrial and organizational psychology*. Routledge.
Heathwood, C. (2019). Which desires are relevant to well-being? *Noûs*. https://doi.org/10.1111/nous.12232
Huang, L., Kern, M.L., Oades, L.G. (2022). *Chinese international students' conceptualizations of wellbeing: A prototype analysis*, Front. Psychol.
Ip, E. C. (2020). The constitutional economics of the World Health Organization. *In Health Econ Policy Law.* https://doi.org/10.1017/S17441331200 00249

Jannarelli, A. (2011). La nuova food insecurity: una prima lettura sistemica. In Rook Basile E., Germanò A. (a cura di) *Agricoltura e insicurezza alimentare, tra crisi della Pac e mercato globale.*

Jannarelli, A. (2015). *Cibi e diritti. Per una agricoltura sostenibile.*

Jarden, A., & Roache, A. (2023). What Is Wellbeing? *International Journal of Environmental Research and Public Health.* https://doi.org/10.3390/ijerph20065006

Kim, H., Doiron, K., Warren, M.A., & Donaldson, S.I. (2018). The international landscape of positive psychology research: A systematic review. In *Int. J. Wellbeing.*

Lanucara, L. (2024) Lo sviluppo culturale sostenibile come modello per costruire il benessere economico-sociale delle comunità. In *Diritto comunitario e degli scambi internazionali* (1–2/2024).

Lee, K. (2009). The World Health Organization (WHO).

Lin, E. (2014). Pluralism about well-being. In *Philosophical Perspectives*, https://www.jstor.org/stable/26614548

Martinón Quintero, R. (2023). Social Sustainability, Agenda 2030 and Human Rights. An Opportunity to Reinforce Economic, Social and Cultural Rights in Developed Countries. In *Ordine internazionale e diritti umani.* ISSN 2284–3531.

Misselbrook, D. (2014). W is for wellbeing and the WHO definition of health. In *British Journal of General Practice.* https://doi.org/10.3399/bjgp14X682381.

Moore, A. (2019). Hedonism. In *The Stanford Encyclopaedia of Philosophy*, Metaphysics Research Lab of the Stanford University.

Pisani, C. (2024). Le nuove frontiere dell'obbligo di sicurezza: l'organizzazione del lavoro tra efficienza e benessere. In *Massimario di giurisprudenza del lavoro*, 4/20249.

Pisciotta Tosini, G. (2025). Animal welfare. In *European and global food law*, III edition.

Rogers, D.S., Duraiappah, A.K., Antons, D.C., Munoz, P., Bai, X., Fragkias. M., & Gutscher, H. (2014). A vision for human well-being: transition to social sustainability. In *Current Opinion in Environmental Sustainability.*

Rusk, R.D., & Water, L.E. (2013). Tracing the size, reach, impact, and breadth of positive psychology. In *J. Posit. Psychol.*

Russo Corvace, G. (2025). Le nuove strategie europee di sostenibilità per il settore Agri-food. In *Teoria* (Teoria 2025/2 n. 46).

Saija, R. (2024). Benessere animale negli allevamenti e protezione durante l'abbattimento. Macellazione rituale e nuove sfide del diritto agroalimentare. In *Rivista di Diritto Alimentare* (3/2024).

Saija, R. (2021). Precauzione e trasparenza del mercato agroalimentare prima e dopo il Covid-19. In *Rivista di Diritto Alimentare* (2/2021).

Saija, R. (2020). Principi di precauzione e sussidiarietà: esiti sul diritto alimentare in tempi di emergenza. In *Rivista di Diritto Alimentare* (2/2020).

Seligman, M.E.P. (2013). *Flourish: A Visionary New Understanding of Happiness and Well-Being*, Simon & Schuster.

Somma, A. (2017). Stato del benessere o benessere dello Stato? Giustizia sociale, politiche demografiche e ordine economico nell'esperienza statunitense. In *Quaderni fiorentini per la storia del pensiero giuridico moderno* (46/2017).

Unanue-Manriquez. W. (2014). *Materialism, personal well-being and environmental behaviour: crossnational and longitudinal evidence from the UK and Chile*, University of Sussex.

Wang, F., Guo, J., & Yang, G. (2023). Study on positive psychology from1999 to 2021: A bibliometric analysis. In *Front. Psychol.*

Yadeun-Antuñano, M., & Vieira, L.C. (2019). Indigenous perspectives of wellbeing: Living a good life. In *Good Health and Well-Being*, Springer International Publishing.

Origin, Evolution, and Scope of the *One Health* Approach in Contemporary Food Law within the Global Context of Climate Change

Gelsomina Russo Corvace

1 Introduction: The Impacts of Climate Change on the Agri-Food Sector

Climate changes, and particularly those that are related to the issue of global warming, are widely discussed nowadays in academics, politics, and the public sphere, given that they are an indisputable reality according to both the Intergovernmental Panel on Climate Change (IPCC) and several other international organizations (Pais et al., 2020, Kumar et al., 2022). In this sense, climate change has often been defined both as a common concern of mankind that can affect populations regardless of state boundaries and as one of the greatest threats to humankind in the twenty-first century (Zhang et al., 2022). An insightful overview of the issue was given by Richard Meserve, president of the Carnegie Institution of Washington and former Chairman of the U.S. Nuclear Regulatory Commission who, while opening a panel

G. R. Corvace (✉)
Campus Bio-Medico University of Rome, Rome, Italy
e-mail: g.russocorvace@unicampus.it

F. Bruno et al. (eds.), *Healthcare and Food*,
https://doi.org/10.1007/978-981-95-5899-5_9

on climate change in 2007, stressed that it is a severe challenge that no one country can solve. On the other hand, Rosina Bierbaum, Dean of the School of Natural Resources and Environment at the University of Michigan, in her analysis of the issue of climate change, stressed the imminent dangers that the world has faced since the beginning of the climate crisis underlying how

> we are not making progress in understanding vulnerability to climate change and its potential impacts on humans, conducting risk analysis or understanding what stakeholders want from science to aid decision making (Bruno et al., 2025).

Climate fluctuations have always caused significant challenges for ecosystems and civilizations. However, in recent years, the phenomenon of climate change has been exacerbated by human activities—first among everything those related to livestock farming, breeding and agriculture—resulting in severe impacts on both the agri-food sector and food security.

In this sense, it is necessary to underline that the global agri-food system comprises *(a)* food production, *(b)* processing, *(c)* packing, *(d)* storage, *(e)* transportation, *(f)* retail, *(g)* consumption, *(h)* loss, and *(i)* waste (Heydari, 2024, Zheng et al., 2024). To be sustainable, the agri-food system is expected to meet the food demand of the present and future generations while maintaining profitability and reducing environmental pollution. Sustainable agri-food production is therefore the origin and prerequisite of the whole agri-food system. Extreme events, such as heat and cold waves, severe droughts and heavy rainfall, stress the vulnerability of the agri-food sector, which is characterized by the peculiarity of producing both positive and negative externalities (Bruno, 2022). The impact of climate change on the agricultural sector, however, varies depending on the farming systems, different in sensitivity and exposure to changes (Salpina et al., 2022).

Food security, on the other hand, is considered to exist when all people, at all times, have physical and economic access to sufficient, safe and nutritious food that meets their dietary needs and preferences, enabling an active and healthy life (as stressed by the World Food

Summit, 1996). Food security is part of a broader framework that further includes food safety, food health, and (more recently), food sustainability. At the European level, the term "food safety" conventionally refers to the hygienic and sanitary safety of food products in terms of health protection, understood in the broadest sense along the entire food chain, and including tools for consumer communication; differently, "food health" refers to the quality of food that goes beyond hygiene requirements and is characterized by the absence of synthetic products or by its ability to enhance individual well-being while "food security," as said, denotes the economic and physical security of having access to sufficient food to meet normal dietary needs (Albisinni, 2023; Benozzo, 2023; Bolognini, 2013). Lastly, "food sustainability" refers to the ability of food systems to ensure long-term food production and distribution in ways that are environmentally sound, economically viable, and socially equitable by preserving natural resources, reducing environmental impacts, and supporting the well-being of current and future generations.

Since food production depends directly on natural resources, which are also closely dependent on climate and weather conditions, increasing food production in a global scenario impacted by climate change is a rather complex challenge, which led experts to think that new agricultural revolutions and transformations might be needed in the near future to ensure equitable access to food for the entire global population (Pais et al., 2020; Reynolds et al., 2010). For instance, the Special Rapporteur on the right to food—a leading international body in the food security field—has highlighted the critical issues of current food systems in terms of greenhouse gas emissions and future food insecurity, calling for the adoption of agroecological and small-scale farming techniques to promote greater sustainability and resilience of systems to climate change, while strengthening food sovereignty. Climate change therefore poses a growing threat to the right to food worldwide (Pitto, 2023, Sage, 2014).

2 Origin and Evolution of the One Health Approach

In response to global food security issues, intended not only as the right to food but also as the right to sustainable food (Brutto, 2025), numerous approaches—especially holistic ones—have emerged in search of a generalized solution. Indeed, in a global context in which the world population has recently exceeded 8 billion and is set to reach around 9.5 billion by 2050, national and supranational legislators are called upon to implement structural regulatory changes to adapt the various global food systems to immediate and future challenges, in an attempt to respond to growing food needs and avert the adverse effects of climate change (Pitto, 2023). Among the most interesting approaches, the ecosystemic, and agroecological ones are certainly worth mentioning as is, for the purpose of the present paper, the "*One Health*" approach.

As expressly stated by the Food and Agriculture Organization of the United Nations (FAO) the "*One Health*" is a methodological, holistic, and multisectoral approach that seeks interdisciplinary solutions to complex challenges (FAO et al., 2023, Bullón Caro, 2025, Bowen, Ebi, 2015). Structured as a multidisciplinary approach based on the awareness of a deep connection between human health, animal health, and environmental health, together with economic, social and cultural factors, "*One Health*" aims to foster collaborative efforts across all sectors (Pitto, 2023, Bullón Caro, 2025, De Gara & Gherardi, 2022) and it has therefore become the subject of study and reflection by international legal doctrine. This derives from the fact that said approach is also applicable to the design and implementation of both programs, policies, and legislation with the aim of achieving better public health outcomes. Furthermore, the interest of legal scholars is justified by the fact that legislation plays a crucial role in the implementation of the paradigm itself. As once again stated by the FAO

> Legislation is a powerful means by which countries and regional organizations translate One Health objectives into concrete, sustainable, and enforceable rights, obligations, and responsibilities (Ragone, 2022, FAO, 2020).

A first formulation of "*One Health*" dates back to 2003 when, in the aftermath of the SARS epidemic, William B. Karesh stated that global health should have to be pursued through a broad approach, based on the awareness that there is only one world and one health. In 2004 said formulation was adopted by the World Conservation Society (WCS) that further published the so-called *Manhattan Principles*, a set of recommendations considered as the scientific manifest of the "*One Health, One World*" concept. Said principles are nothing more than the result of discussions held by a group of human and animal health experts who gathered at Rockefeller University in New York. In this sense, they are aimed at promoting an international and multidisciplinary approach to health protection, based on the abovementioned recognition of the interconnections between human and animal medicine and health (Bullón Caro, 2025, De Gara & Gherardi, 2022, Pitto, 2023 Ragone, 2022). The idea that the two disciplines are closely interconnected is, after all, very old. Among the first luminaries of this vision there are Rudolf Virchow, who discovered zoonoses, and Calvin Schwabe, the progenitor of veterinary epidemiology, who coined the term "*One Medicine*" precisely to emphasize that there is no continuity between human and veterinary medicine (Ragone, 2022, Zinsstag et al., 2021).

A key tenet of the "*One Health*" approach has been the inclusion of all relevant stakeholders, from conceptualizing and planning through implementation and assessment of the "*One Health*" activities which can be defined as

> any research, policy development and implementation, capacity and infrastructure development, and system building or strengthening activities relevant to the health and well-being of humans, animals, plants, or ecosystems (Mumford et al., 2023).

Since its adoption, the approach has been promoted by several intergovernmental organizations, while still relatively nascent and theoretical, with the aim of encouraging intersectoral and multidisciplinary collaboration. Through widening use and the availability of experience and best practices, the "*One Health*" approach evolved, matured, and became more robust (Mumford et al., 2023) eventually reaching a comprehensive definition in 2021, proposed by the One Health High-Level Expert Panel (OHHLEP). More specifically, the definition states that "*One Health*" approach is:

> an integrated, unifying approach that aims to sustainably balance and optimize the health of people, animals and ecosystems. It recognizes that the health of humans, domestic and wild animals, plants, and the wider environment (including ecosystems) are closely linked and interdependent. The approach mobilizes multiple sectors, disciplines and communities at varying levels of society to work together to foster well-being and tackle threats to health and ecosystems. It addresses the collective need for clean water, energy and air, and safe and nutritious food, promoting action on climate change and contributing to sustainable development.

Prior to the adoption of OHHLEP's definition of "*One Health,*" there were multiple ones coexisting together, each emphasizing different aspects of the approach (Abbas et al., 2022, Bullón Caro, 2025b, Nzietchueng et al., 2023).

> Said lack of definitional consistency hindered the development of a coherent, science-based framework for integrating One Health into legal and policy frameworks. A unified definition is essential for conceptualizing and characterizing One Health from a legal perspective, as only a clearly articulated and broadly accepted concept can be unambiguously incorporated into broader legal and policy instruments. Recognizing this need, OHHLEP prioritized the development of a comprehensive definition, adopting a non-anthropocentric perspective and promoting equity across all sectors. This definition has garnered support from the Quadripartite [...] and is frequently referenced by scholars, [...] regional [...] and international organizations (Bullón Caro, 2025b).

Just by considering the multitude of sources in which the concept of "*One Health*" is now examined and embedded it is possible to understand the importance that its implementation has in decision-making processes (Leone, 2025). As stated, when it comes to "*One Health's*" implementation legislation is crucial. In fact, well-crafted laws and regulations, supported by effective enforcement mechanisms, have the potential to sustain multisectoral and multidisciplinary collaboration even when the initial enthusiasm fades, ensuring long-term sustainability (Bullón Caro, 2025, FAO, 2020). By delineating clear roles and responsibilities for both public and private stakeholders, legislation establishes an accountability framework that is conducive to effective implementation. However, it is inevitable that when legal experts confront the approach, they question its essence, implications and legal ramifications, leading to significant questions on its legal nature, substantive content, obligations, and enforcement/implementation mechanisms (Bullón Caro, 2025). Nonetheless, various elements of the accepted OHHLEP's definition provide guidance into understanding and incorporating "*One Health*" into legislation.

> The first part of the definition underlines the need for a unifying approach across sectors and disciplines, seeking to balance regulatory objectives traditionally addressed in isolation. The second part emphasizes multisectoral and multidisciplinary collaboration as a defining element of One Health, along with whole-of-society approaches. As integral components of the definition, these elements are intrinsic to the concept itself: One Health necessitates active stakeholder engagement, a cross-sectoral focus, and a commitment to sustainable development. The final part of the definition positions the environment as a collective necessity, advocating for its legal protection and integration into policymaking. It further presents One Health as a pathway to sustainable development, fostering multisectoral collaboration to balance environmental, social, and economic considerations (Bullón Caro, 2025b).

In addition to the formal definition, OHHLEP has identified five fundamental principles of "*One Health*" which can be summarized in *(i)* equity between sectors *(ii)* socio-political and multicultural parity, *(iii)* socioecological equilibrium to reach harmonious balance between humans, animals and the environment, *(iv)* stewardship and the responsibility of humans to change behavior and adopt sustainable solutions with regard to both animal welfare, ecosystems and future generations, and lastly *(v)* transdisciplinary and multisectoral collaboration, in relation to all relevant modern and traditional disciplines. As a matter of fact, when it comes to the legal sector the "*One Health*" approach encompasses a variety of legal fields, including both environmental and agricultural law, generally regulated separately. This makes the incorporation of the approach into legislation harder, requiring solutions that are adaptable to the specific legal issue or area involved (Bullón Caro, 2025b).

The European Union, for instance, is deploying "*One Health*" principles across multiple areas and sectors increasing its use over the years. With specific reference to legal acts, the "*One Health*" approach is mentioned in 8 Regulations, 1 Directive (no longer in force), 7 Decisions, and as many as 22 Communications (Coli & Schebesta, 2023). While at the beginning "*One Health*" was only confined to Antimicrobial Resistance (AMR) and zoonoses control, it has now stretched beyond the fields of animal welfare, biodiversity, soil health, sustainable use of pesticides, climate and health, prevention, detection, and rapid response to future health emergencies. Among the most significant initiatives we can find: 1. the Farm to Fork Strategy; 2. the adoption of Regulations (EU) 2022/2371 (on serious cross-border threats to health), (EU) 2022/2370 (on the establishment of European Centre for Disease Prevention and Control—ECDC) and (EU) 2022/123 (on the European Medicines Agency—EMA); 3. the European Health Emergency Preparedness and Response Authority (HERA), created in 2021 to prevent, detect, and rapidly respond to health emergencies, including AMR-related threats and other potential crises; and 4. the Global Health Strategy of 2022. Before the adoption of the Green Deal, we had first encountered the term "*One Health*" across EU law in 2010, where reference was only made to "the concept of one world, one health."

> Indeed, at that time, One Health was not perceived as an autonomous concept untethered from the Manhattan Principles [...] instead, it appeared at best as an "initiative" of the international arena. Moreover, the European Commission recognized One Health as expressing the unique link between human and animal health, not considering environmental health. Years later, the 2017 EU One Health Action Plan Against AMR was launched as a cornerstone of the One Health policy framework at the European level. It represented a turning point for at least four reasons: a) it includes the first ever definition of One Health provided by the EU. The definition is noteworthy because it states that "the One Health

approach also encompasses the environment" (italics added), which is only acknowledged as a link between humans and animals and as a source of new resistant microorganisms. Thus, the European Commission did not consider the three dimensions of One Health on the same level, instead adopting a rather intensely anthropocentric perspective that does not take into account the environment; b) despite the narrow and likely inadequate formulation of the One Health definition, the Action Plan contains some remarks worth mentioning since they express the need to broaden One Health's scope. The document states, surprisingly, that "initiatives need to be broadened, for example by extending the One Health approach to include the environment" and considers AMR as a "good example of a One Health matter". Thus, AMR is considered only as one of several issues where the approach is worth applying, paving the way to a wider understanding of One Health; c) it correlates One Health with policy coherence, introducing the term in the context of policy-making; d) it refers to One Health both as a "principle" and an "approach", giving it greater legitimacy than in the past, where it was acknowledged as an "initiative" or "concept" (Coli & Schebesta, 2023).

After the adoption of the Green Deal, "*One Health*" has been fully recognized as a horizontal and fundamental principle encompassing all EU policies finally reaching a harmonious dynamic among its three dimensions (i.e., humans, animals, and the planet) and becoming a key tool to be taken into consideration by both policymakers and judicial bodies with regard to their legal interpretation.

Nevertheless, even though from a legal standpoint the "*One Health*" approach is reaching a high level of implementation, it still seems to be a prerogative of natural sciences which are certainly the primarily responsible for its origin, and it seems clear that as of today they can be further considered the major contributors to its active development. Indeed, while the use of the "*One Health*" concept has increased, the increase is mostly driven by the sectors of human and veterinary medicine and the most active "*One Health*" scholars, are from the field of veterinary research (Humboldt-Dachroeden et al., 2020). Therefore, it is essential to take advantage of the current momentum to move forward with the "*One Health*" approach, especially in the legal field (i.e., food law, environmental law etc.), where different yet interconnected solutions are required.

3 The One Health Approach as a Driver for Combating Climate Change and Preserving Biodiversity, Ecosystems, and Access to Food

> The "*One Health*" ideas of today constitute a reconceptualization of health management in response to the exponentially accelerating environmental changes of the past 100 years associated with the parallel exponential growth of the global human population. The number of people on earth, the intensity of our activities and the pace and extent of environmental change have never been as great as they are today (Evans & Leighton, 2014).

The usefulness of the "*One Health*" approach with regard to global climate change and its impacts especially on food systems can be seen when considering that climate change is characterized by disruptions in the geographical distribution of infectious diseases, due to changes in the spread of pathogen-related animals and insects. As a matter of fact, from a "*One Health*" perspective, climate change can have considerable impact on factors that may affect disease transmission such as spatial distribution of vectors, encroachment into animal habitats, disruption of animal migration pathways and altered behavior and management by communities of animals, crops and their environments. In addition, there is a direct impact on human, animal, and environmental health resulting from extreme weather events, drought, and rising average temperatures, and their consequences on the nutritional levels of the food we consume (Pitto, 2023, Zhang et al., 2022).

In this sense, it is therefore clear that the two sectors with the strongest links to health risks due to climate change effects are: *(i)* the agri-food sector (Russo Corvace, 2025), as a result of threats to the yield, quality, and affordability of food stock and the resultant impacts on undernutrition, and *(ii)* the water sector, due to the risks related to water-borne and food-borne diseases. Access and right to food—as mentioned in paragraph 2—are other sectors where climate fluctuations have significant implications, with rising sea levels posing challenges to agriculture and increasing temperatures leading to land degradation and agricultural failures (Shafique et al., 2024). Effectively preparing for and managing these and other risks requires systems-based approaches that address the multiple drivers of adverse health outcomes (Bowen, Ebi 2015). While slowing down climate change is a certain priority, adaptation to the changing climate and trying to do the best to protect humans, animals, and shared environments from its negative impacts are an even more urgent need. It is evident that human health is intimately related to the health of our surrounding environments, including animals and plants, and to the ecosystems on which all of us depend. In this sense, the "*One Health*" approach is deemed as one of the best solutions to achieve optimal health and well-being outcomes (De Gara & Gherardi, 2022, Zhang et al., 2022, Zinnstag et al., 2020) since, in an increasingly interconnected world, where the journey from farm to fork goes through multiple sectors, it recognizes that both food safety and security need a multidisciplinary, sustainable and collaborative approach. Foodborne illnesses, a pressing global concern, often stem from the convergence of human, animal, and environmental factors, while pathogens can emerge from livestock, wildlife, or contaminated water sources, infiltrating the food chain and affecting both humans and animals. Indeed, "*One Health*" initiatives bolster surveillance and response systems, enabling early detection of potential foodborne outbreaks. By promoting collaboration between the agriculture, veterinary, and public health sectors, the approach can help identify and mitigate food safety risks, ensuring access to safe and nutritious food for all (Danasekaran, 2024, FAO, 2018).

> Without being exhaustive, a "*One Health*" approach to climate change may significantly contribute to the following contexts and issues: food security with particular emphasis on animal source foods, extensive livestock systems, especially the role of ruminant livestock, antimicrobial resistance control, environmental sanitation, and steps towards regional

and global integrated syndromic surveillance and response systems (Zinsstag et al., 2018).

According to the World Food Summit, as mentioned under paragraph 1, food security exists when all people, at all times, have physical and economic access to sufficient, safe, and nutritious food that meets their dietary needs and preferences, enabling an active, and healthy life. A more recent approach to food security stresses not only the material access to food, but the need for it to be sustainable, in a way that helps preserve ecosystems and the environment as whole. In this context, significant impacts of climate change on agriculture and food security are a relatively new reality, making it imperative that farmers, shepherds, fisheries, and forest sectors and enterprises can gain access to new technologies, markets, information and credit to adjust their production management systems and practices (Pais et al., 2020) to a new sustainable and holistic approach. Health is an essential component of the capacity to adapt to climate change (Berry et al., 2011). On the other hand, AMR is a major global health crisis characterized by the ability of microorganisms—bacteria, viruses, fungi, and parasites—to survive antimicrobial treatments that were previously effective against them. The World Health Organization (WHO) classifies AMR as one of the greatest threats to human health, with resistant infections causing approximately 700.000 deaths annually—a figure projected to rise to 10 million per year by 2050 without an urgent intervention. As much as guaranteeing food security, effectively addressing the threats of AMR—mostly caused by the negative impacts of climate change—requires integrated mitigation and adaptation strategies rooted in the "*One Health*" approach (Alhassan & Ahmad, 2025).

Since climate change and its associated health burdens do not strike evenly, they tend to exacerbate existing inequities in access to safe and nutritious food. A "*One Health*" interpretation of the right to food—as advanced in recent doctrine—requires that States secure not only availability and access to food itself, but also sustainability of the diets offered, meaning that they must ensure products that are of high quality, produced with non-invasive practices and beneficial for the health of humans (Brutto, 2025). This supports measures that privilege new techniques and agroecological practices, small-scale producers and knowledge systems capable of pushing away climatic shocks, while "internalizing externalities" that have historically been socialized (i.e., environmental degradation, public-health costs of AMR). In other words, "*One Health*" thus channels the progressive realization of the right to food toward a model of sustainable food systems that are consistent with planetary boundaries and more local centered approaches.

While animal health, human health and environmental health are intricately linked, our approach to understanding health risks is still mostly independent. The needed collaboration and communication across and between scientific disciplines has been lacking or non-existent. "*One Health*" advances a sustained partnership across disciplines and has been demonstrating accomplishments in tackling complex health risks (Ruscio et al., 2015). In addition, it invites us to face head on the limits of anthropocentrism and to interrogate the possibility that the complex, often beautiful ecosystems on which we depend have a value that exceeds their human usefulness (Sheather, 2023).

4 Conclusion: The Road toward Mitigation and Adaptation

The "*One Health*" approach is becoming way more than a scientific narrative. It is also a legal method for governing climate-related risks and steering food systems toward resilience and justice. By insisting on the interdependence of human, animal and environmental health, "*One Health*" reframes classic food-law objectives (i.e., the traditional concepts of food safety, food security, and food health) within an integrated structure capable of addressing complex, global harms intensified by climate change. In legal terms, this means elevating coordination duties, mainstreaming precaution and prevention, and operationalizing accountability across sectors and jurisdictions. In this context, food security—as articulated since the Rome Declaration and further specified by contemporary doctrine—cannot be secured without simultaneously ensuring food safety, food health (intended here as nutritional adequacy), and food sustainability. The four dimensions rise or fall together, particularly when extreme weather and ecological degradation affect yields, quality and affordability, and when zoonotic dynamics and antimicrobial resistance (AMR) travel along agroecological interfaces. The law therefore cannot treat these concerns separately: it must require joined-up risk governance that acts at source, along the chain, and at interfaces with water, soil, and wildlife. The OHHLEP definition provides a normative standpoint of the paradigm. By describing "*One Health*" as an «integrated, unifying approach» that aims to «sustainably balance and optimize» the health of people, animals, and ecosystems, it legitimates a non-anthropocentric perspective and a program of equity, stewardship, and trans-disciplinarity (De Gara & Gherardi, 2022, Zinsstag et al., 2020). With regard to positive law, those principles translate into legislative and governmental choices: multisectoral mandates, interoperable surveillance, and cooperation that bind both public authorities and market operators. In other words, "*One Health*" moves the law from a sector-based logic to a more proactive and system-level one aimed at anticipating, monitoring, sharing data, and mitigating climate change-related risks.

The European Union experience confirms the abovementioned evolution of the "*One Health*" approach. While initially anchored in AMR and zoonoses control, "*One Health*" has in fact been progressively deployed across food, veterinary medicines, environmental and emergency-preparedness regimes, now expressly governing Green Deal strategies and the Farm to Fork objectives. Instruments such as the 2017 "*One Health*" Action Plan against AMR, the post-2020 health-security package (including the reinforced mandates of ECDC and EMA) and the establishment of HERA demonstrate how general principles are being embedded in concrete competences, workflows, and metrics. The EU now recognizes "*One Health*" as horizontal to Union action and relevant for judicial interpretation and administrative enforcement.

This evolution carries several implications. Firstly, "*One Health*" strengthens the principle of integration: when regulating on agriculture, veterinary medicines, pesticides, or consumer information, institutions must weigh effects on human, animal, and ecosystem health as interconnected variables, not externalities. This has consequences for impact assessments and the allocation of burdens of proof under the precautionary principle in conditions of scientific uncertainty. Secondly, it reframes due diligence across public and private actors: producers, veterinarians, feed manufacturers, laboratories, and retailers share a duty to prevent and reduce risks that are foreseeable across sectors (as for example, resistance emergence from inappropriate antimicrobial use, contamination via water or wildlife vectors). Lastly, it supports policy coherence by aligning food-law choices with climate, biodiversity, and public-health strategies, avoiding the well-documented oscillation between productivity maximization and downstream risk management.

From the analysis developed in the present paper it therefore emerges that an integrated surveillance and governance of data is needed, meaning that legislation should mandate interoperable monitoring of zoonoses, residues, and environmental matrices across the food chain (Bowen & Ebi, 2015, Danasekaran, 2024), with shared indicators and timely data that flows between food safety, veterinary, and environmental authorities. Where uncertainty persists, legislative provisions should authorize preventive restrictions that are proportionate to potential global harms. Such approach may reduce the lag between ecological signals and administrative action. Climate adaptation in food law further requires diversification of production, infrastructure for safe storage and transport under extreme weather, and contingency protocols that protect vulnerable consumers from supply disruptions without compromising safety or nutrition. Legislative frameworks should recognize ecosystem services as part of the food-law sector enabling payments for ecological performance and liability for degradation that foreseeably undermines food security. Additionally, Councils, Centers and Authorities created or repurposed with "*One Health*" mandates—from ECDC/EMA to HERA—can coordinate complex portfolios when they are given clear legal bases, explicit data-access powers, and evaluation duties that are tied to "*One Health*" indicators. In this sense, judicial review plays a crucial and complementary role in assessing whether administrations respected precaution and prevention and allocated burdens fairly across the chain. In turn, private-law instruments (contractual clauses or certification schemes) can diffuse "*One Health*" due diligence expectations downstream to retailers and upstream to input suppliers.

The ethics of the "*One Health*" approach also carries legal weight. If ecosystems have value beyond their immediate utility to humans, as argued by recent commentators, then proportionality analyses must recognize ecological integrity as an independent interest, not a mere substitute for human welfare. This has practical effects: for instance, in calibrating pesticide approvals, intensive operations, or balancing emergency derogations during shortages, the least harmful alternative must be assessed holistically, not through a narrow, single-risk lens.

Finally, this paper's cross-reading of climate impacts, food system vulnerabilities and the evolution of "*One Health*" suggests a research and policy agenda. Legislators should not only conduct "*One Health*" legal audits of the existing food chain legislation to identify fragmentation or contradictory incentives but also integrate "*One Health*" impact assessments into new proposals, resource joint surveillance infrastructures and laboratory capacity and incorporate equity safeguards so that adaptation and mitigation measures do not shift risks to low-income producers or consumers. Said goals are expressions of a constitutional duty, both national and supranational, to secure a high level of health protection and to ensure coherent, science-informed governance in the face of transboundary, climate change-related risks.

In conclusion, the "*One Health*" approach sets forth new interpretative directives for contemporary food law in the Anthropocene/climate change era. It translates the insight of interdependence into concrete duties of cooperation, prevention, and stewardship. Further, it aligns the right to food with sustainability, and it equips courts and administrations with criteria for proportionate, evidence-sensitive decisions under uncertainty. With the correct level of integration into legislative and institutional provisions "*One Health*" can turn the dual track of mitigation and adaptation to climate changes into a coherent program of integral well-being (*see* Bruno, Brutto in the present volume) for people, animals and ecosystems, making the food system not merely a sector to be defended from climate impacts, but a lever for transformative and lawful change.

References

Abbas, S., Shorten, T., & Rushton, J. (2022). Meanings and mechanisms of one health partnerships: Insights from a critical review of literature on cross government collaborations. *Health Policy and Planning, 37*(3), 385–399. https://doi.org/10.1093/heapol/czab134

Albisinni, F. (2023). *Le declinazioni della sicurezza alimentare. Strumentario di diritto alimentare europeo.* Wolters Kluwer.

Alhassan, M.Y., & Ahmad, A.A. (2025). Antimicrobial resistance in a changing climate: a One Health approach for adaptation and mitigation. *Bulletin of the National Research Centr*e, *49*, 26. https://doi.org/10.1186/s42269-025-01318-2.

Benozzo, M. (2023). *Biotecnologie agroalimentari e nuove tecniche di miglioramento genetico tra Unione Europea e Stati Uniti*. Aracne.

Berry, H. L., Hogan, A., Ng, S. P., & Parkinson, A. (2011). Farmer health and adaptive capacity in the face of climate change and variability. Part 1: Health as a contributor to adaptive capacity and as an outcome from pressures coping with climate related adversities. *International Journal of Environmental Research and Public Health, 8*, 4039–4054. https://doi.org/10.3390/ijerph8104039

Bolognini, S. (2013). Food safety e comunicazione ai cittadini in materia di sicurezza e di rischio alimentari: il concetto di prodotto alimentare insicuro al vaglio della Corte di giustizia, *Riv. dir. agr., 2013, II, 93-119*, (ISSN: 0391-8696).

Bowen, K. J., & Ebi, K. L. (2015). Governing the health risks of climate change: Towards multi-sector responses. *Current Opinion in Environmental Sustainability, 12*, 80–85. https://doi.org/10.1016/j.cosust.2014.12.001

Bruno, F. (2022). *Il Diritto Alimentare, sviluppo sostenibile e tutela della salute.* Wolters Kluwer (CEDAM).

Bruno, F., & Russo Corvace, G., (2025). Environment and climate change. European and Global Food Law (3d ed., pp. 420–433).

Brutto, G. (2025). Diritto al cibo e diritto ad un cibo sostenibile. *Teoria* 2025/2 n. 46.

Bullón Caro, C. (2025). One health, sustainable development and the principle of integration: Legal synergies for effective implementation. *Research Directions: One Health., 3*(e5), 1–10. https://doi.org/10.1017/one.2025.1

Bullón Caro, C. (2025b). Legal elements to operationalise one health: From principles to practice. *Research Directions: One Health.*, *3*(e4), 1–11. https://doi.org/10.1017/one.2025.2

Coli, F., & Schebesta, H. (2023). One health in the EU: The next future? *European Papers, 8*(1), 301–316. https://doi.org/10.15166/2499-8249/652

Danasekaran, R. (2024). One health: A holistic approach to tackling Global Health issues. *Indian Journal of Community Medicine, 49*, 260–263. https://doi.org/10.4103/ijcm.ijcm_521_23

De Gara, L., & Gherardi M. (2022). Modelli di analisi con metodologie innovative del rischio di esposizione ad agenti chimici e biologici in agricoltura in ottica "one health". *Rivista degli infortuni e delle malattie professionali* (2/2022).

Evans, B. R., & Leighton, F. A. (2014). A history of one health. *Rev. sci. tech. Off. int. Epiz., 33*(2), 413–420.

Food and Agriculture Organization (FAO), World Organization for Animal Health (OIE), World Health Organization (WHO). (2018). *Taking a multisectoral, one health approach: A tripartite guide to addressing zoonotic diseases in countries*. FAO.

Food and Agriculture Organization of the United Nations (FAO). (2020). *One Health legislation: Contributing to pandemic prevention through law*. Retrieved from https://openknowledge.fao.org/items/2c552824-4729-4050-9cb6-4557580812e6

Food and Agriculture Organization of the United Nations (FAO), United Nations Environmental Programme (UNEP), World Health Organization (WHO) and World Animal Health Organisation (WOAH) (2023). *A guide to implementing of the one health joint plan of action at national level*. Retrieved from https://openknowledge.fao.org/items/d5be526e-36a6-4c90-8b7c-75ac01bc340c

Heydari, M. (2024). Cultivating sustainable global food supply chains: A multifaceted approach to mitigating food loss and waste for climate resilience. *J Cleaner Production.*, *442*(October 2023), 141037. https://doi.org/10.1016/j.jclepro.2024.141037

Humboldt-Dachroeden, S., Rubin, O., & Sylvester Frid-Nielsen, S. (2020). The state of one health research across disciplines and sectors—a bibliometric analysis. *One Health, 10*(2020), 100146. https://doi.org/10.1016/j.onehlt.2020.100146

Kumar, L., Chhogyel, N., Gopalakrishnan, T., Hasan, M. K., Jayasinghe, S. L., Kariyawasam, C. S., Kipkemboi Kogo, B., & Ratnayake, S. (2022). Climate change and future of Agri-food production. In *Future foods* (pp. 49–79). Academic Press. https://doi.org/10.1016/B978-0-323-91001-9.00009-8

Leone, L. (2025). L'approccio One Health nella legislazione europea sugli animali: orientamenti e prospettive. *Rivista Eurojus, Fascicolo, 1-2025*, 163–186.

Mumford, E. L., Martinez, D. J., Tyance-Hassell, K., Cook, A., et al. (2023). Evolution and expansion of the one health approach to promote sustainable and resilient health and well-being: A call to action. *Frontiers in Public Health*. https://doi.org/10.3389/fpubh.2022.1056459

Nzietchueng, S., Kitua, A., Nyatanyi, T., & Rwego, I. B. (2023). Facilitating implementation of the one health approach: A definition of a one health intervention. *One Health, 16*, 100491. https://doi.org/10.1016/j.onehlt.2023.100491

Pais, I. P., Reboredo, F. H., Ramalho, J. C., Pessoa, M. F., Lidon, F. C., & Silva, M. M. (2020). Potential impacts of climate change on agriculture—a review. *Emirates Journal of Food and Agriculture., 32*(6), 397–407. https://doi.org/10.9755/ejfa.2020.v32.i6.2111

Pitto, S. (2023). Cambiamento climatico e sicurezza alimentare: dall'approccio *One Health* ai modelli del *Global South*. BioLaw Journal—Rivista di BioDiritto, (2), 315–47. https://doi.org/10.15168/2284-4503-2712

Ragone, G. (2022). One Health e Costituzione italiana, tra spinte eco-centriche e nuove prospettive di tutela della salute umana, ambientale e animale. One World, One Health... Which law? *Corti supreme e salute, 3*, 809–826.

Reynolds, C., Crompton, L., & Mills, J. (2010). Livestock and climate change impacts in the developing world. *Outlook on Agriculture, 39*, 245–248. https://doi.org/10.5367/oa.2010.0015

Ruscio, B. A., Brubaker, M., Glasser, J., Hueston, W., & Hennessy, T. W. (2015). One health—A strategy for resilience in a changing arctic. *International Journal of Circumpolar Health, 2015*(74), 27913. https://doi.org/10.3402/ijch.v74.27913

Russo Corvace, G. (2025). New European sustainability strategies for the Agri-food sector. *Teoria* 2025/2 n. 46.

Sage, C. (2014). Food security, food sovereignty and the special rapporteur. Shaping food policy discourse through realizing the right to food. *Dialogues in Human Geography, 4*, 195.

Salpina, D., & Pagliacci, F. (2022). Are we adapting to climate change? Evidence from the high-quality Agri-food sector in the Veneto region. *Sustainability, 14*, 11482. https://doi.org/10.3390/su141811482

Shafique, M., Kurshid, M., Muzammil, S., Arshad, M.I., Malik, I.R., Rasool, M.H., Khalid, A., Khalid, R., Asghar, R., Baloch, Z. and Aslam, B. (2024). Traversed dynamics of climate change and One Health. *Environmental Sciences Europe, 36*, 135. https://doi.org/10.1186/s12302-024-00931-8.

Sheater, J. (2023). One health and climate change—We need to get the ethics right. *BMJ, 383*, p2177. https://doi.org/10.1136/bmj.p2177

World Food Summit. (1996). *Rome Declaration on World Food Security.* 13–17 November, World Food Summit, Rome.

Zhang, R., Tang, X., Liu, J. (2022). From concept to action: a united, holistic and One Health approach to respond to the climate change crisis. *Infectious Diseases of Poverty, 11*, 17. doi:https://doi.org/10.1186/s40249-022-00941-9.

Zheng, H., Ma, W., & Zhou, X. (2024). Promoting sustainable agrifood production under climate change: Adaptation, returns, and food security implications. *International Journal of Sustainable Development & World Ecology, 31*(8), 1083–1094. https://doi.org/10.1080/13504509.2024.2385095

Zinsstag, J., Crump, L., Schelling, E. et al. (2018). Climate change and One Health, FEMS Microbiology Letters. 365, fny085. https://doi.org/10.1093/femsle/fny085.

Zinsstag, J., Schelling, E., Crump, L., Whittaker, M., Tanner, M., & Stephen, C. (2020). *One health: The theory and practice of integrated health approaches.* CAB International.

Zinsstag, J., Waltner-Toews, D., Tanner, M. (2021). Why one health? One health: The theory and practice of integrated health approaches. CAB International (II ed.)

Food Systems Challenges Between Tradition and New Technologies

Camilla Clerici

1 Introduction: the Challenges Faced by Food Systems

Food systems in the twenty-first century are undergoing a period of profound transformation to address the growing environmental, demographic and economic challenges that have demonstrated the unsustainability of agricultural and food production models. In fact, in recent decades, climate and biodiversity crises, intensive exploitation of natural and animal resources, and unstoppable population growth have led key European and international players to redesign environmental, food, economic and social policies.

According to United Nations projections, the world population is estimated to reach ten billion by 2050, which will lead to an increase in food demand of about 60% compared to current levels. As a result, food systems will need to be able to guarantee sufficient food supplies for the

C. Clerici (✉)
Campus Bio-Medico University of Rome, Rome, Italy
e-mail: camilla.clerici@hotmail.it

F. Bruno et al. (eds.), *Healthcare and Food*,
https://doi.org/10.1007/978-981-95-5899-5_10

entire population while meeting high food safety standards and generating the least possible impact on the environment (Choudhury et al., 2020).

Said global context led the latest international and European entities and strategies to guide the transition towards more sustainable models. For instance, the United Nations 2030 Agenda defines 17 Sustainable Development Goals (SDGs), including Zero Hunger and food security, combating climate change, protecting ecosystems and promoting sustainable models (Castellani et al., 2025).

At the same time, EU legislation has proposed an agricultural model capable of integrating economic considerations with sustainability over time and compatibility with the territory, the environment and society. This objective is made even clearer and more pressing by both the document on the Common Agricultural Policy (CAP) for 2020, the approval of the Green Deal (2019) and the related From Farm to Fork strategy. Those are the policy documents with which the European Union intends to achieve the goal of zero emissions by 2050, for which a massive transformation of the agricultural sector, land use and production processes will be essential. In particular, in the From Farm to Fork strategy, the Commission reaffirms its commitment by stating that

> current food consumption patterns are unsustainable from both health and environmental points of view. (...) Tackling food loss and waste is key to achieving sustainability. Reducing food waste ties in with policies on the recovery of nutrients and secondary raw materials, the production of feed, food safety, biodiversity, bioeconomy, waste management and renewable energy.

In light of this, the Commission has committed itself for the coming years to presenting, among other things, legislative proposals aimed at reducing dependence on raw materials in the livestock sector (particularly for animal feed) and promoting alternative sources of nutrients. With specific regard to meat, given the desire and need to reduce overall consumption, the European strategy aims to decrease the carbon footprint of livestock farming by every means possible, including (and, one might say, primarily) technological innovation, using food biotechnology. According to the data available as of today, the latter are considered to be an effective and sustainable solution to the problems of sustainability and access to food, animal welfare, and the prevention and reduction of health risks for the population linked to livestock production.

Technical and scientific progress could therefore be a key factor in achieving these objectives (IFLA 2019): the use of New Genomic Techniques (NGTs), Genetically Modified Organisms (GMOs) and Novel Foods could help—together with digitalization—to support a green and digital transition in the agri-food sector.

In this context, the development of cell culture technologies and their application in the production of alternatives to animal proteins has the potential to reduce the negative impacts of traditional livestock farming. Several studies have shown that cultivated meat would reduce the use of water, land and soil, generating benefits in terms of biodiversity preservation, protection of natural habitats and, above all, reduction of greenhouse gases.

In any case, the studies conducted so far are based on projections or limited data, due to the small market share occupied by cultivated meat and the absence of large-scale distribution of such products. This makes it difficult to accurately predict the environmental impact of new production methods, especially in the long term, as well as their ability to create a more sustainable food system (Chriki & Hocquette, 2020).

In addition to environmental considerations, the potential of cultivated meat must also be assessed based on other relevant factors, such as the possible positive effects in combating antibiotic resistance, the spread of animal diseases and the promotion of animal welfare. For these reasons, this new type of meat has also been called "slaughter-free meat" or "clean meat", to highlight the revolutionary nature of these production methods, which do not involve the death of animals and reduce environmental impacts (Lanzoni et al., 2024; Post et al., 2020).

However, despite these positive aspects, discussions and debates on cultivated meat are highly controversial, as the scientific community has reiterated the need for further studies to conclude on food safety profiles. The Food and Agriculture Organization (FAO) has published a detailed report urging private and public actors to investigate potential critical issues for consumer health, such as biological risks and risks related to the type of culture, chemical contaminants and allergenicity (FAO-WHO, 2023).

Moreover, beyond food safety issues, the debate is fueled by socio-economic, cultural and ethical questions, particularly regarding the effects that the spread of cultured meat may have on traditional culinary products or food production methods, which are often linked to the preservation of national identity. On the other hand, additional considerations arise regarding workers in the traditional meat and livestock sectors, as well as the fact that only a few large companies have the tools and knowledge necessary to develop such innovative foods, and therefore the potential positive effects on the world population are undoubtedly limited (Mancini & Antonioli, 2022a, 2022b).

In Italy, for instance, the legislator has taken a strict stance, banning the production, marketing, import and export of food and feed consisting of, isolated from or produced from cell cultures or tissues derived from vertebrate animals, with the aim of protecting human health and the interests of citizens, as well as preserving the agri-food heritage, «as a set of products that express Italy's socio-economic and cultural evolution and are of strategic importance to the national interest». Beyond the legal and technical reasons and legitimacy on which this ban is based, the law highlights the deep connection between national identity and the Country's culinary tradition, further protected by a series of national legislative provisions that protect traditional agri-food products and which, in addition to being governed by ad hoc provisions, are also exempt from European rules on hygiene, premises and materials used.

The Italian case can be considered emblematic in illustrating the polarization of the debate surrounding new technologies applied in the food sector, which complicates the regulation of the matter by European legislators and policymakers, who must consider numerous interests and rights while ensuring maximum protection of human health and the free movement of goods.

2 New Food Technologies: Regulatory Profiles and the Cell-Based Meat

In recent years, within the European Union, cultured meat has been the subject of numerous economic, political and regulatory considerations, which have led to ambiguous and still evolving results.

From a regulatory point of view, cultivated meat falls within the scope of Regulation (EU) 2015/2283 (i.e., Regulation (EU) 2015/2283 of the European Parliament and of the Council of 25 November 2015 on novel foods, amending Regulation (EU) No 1169/2011 of the European Parliament and of the Council and repealing Regulation (EC) No 258/97 of the European Parliament and of the Council and Commission Regulation (EC) No 1852/2001) governing so-called "Novel Foods", which are defined as foods that have not been used for human consumption to a significant degree within the Union before 15 May 1997 (temporal criterion) and that, at the same time, belong to one of the categories listed in Art. 3(2)a, in particular no. iv), which concerns «food consisting of, isolated from or produced from cell culture or tissue culture derived from animals». Furthermore, if GMOs are also used in the production of said foods, the relevant regulatory framework must also apply (which is Directive 2011/18/EC on contained use in agriculture, Regulations (EC) No. 1829/2003 and No. 1830/2003 on GMO foods and feed, as well as on their traceability and labelling) (Seehafer & Bartles, 2019).

The Novel Foods Regulation complements Regulation (EC) No 178/2002 by providing for a very strict preventive control system, which is prior to marketing and consumption. This is clear from Recital 20, which states that:

> novel foods should be authorised and used only if they fulfil the criteria laid down in this Regulation. Novel foods should be safe and if their safety cannot be assessed and scientific uncertainty persists, the precautionary principle may be applied. Their use should not mislead the consumer. Therefore, where a novel food is intended to replace another food, it should not differ from that food in a way that would be nutritionally less advantageous for the consumer.

and, with reference to the role of the Union, Recital 42:

> since the objectives of this Regulation, in particular the laying down of rules for the placing of novel foods on the market within the Union, cannot be sufficiently achieved by the Member States but can rather be better achieved at Union level, the Union may adopt measures, in accordance with the principle of subsidiarity as set out in Article 5 TEU. In accordance with the principle of proportionality, as set out in that Article, this Regulation does not go beyond what is necessary in order to achieve those objectives.

In addition, the Regulation lays down a specific procedure for the inclusion of a food in the list of novel foods and its placing on the market (Articles 6 and 7), as well as specific alert measures for the placing on the market of unauthorized foods. In particular, Article 7 identifies the conditions under which a food may be included among novel foods and subsequently marketed. This occurs if, and only if, it meets the following conditions:

> (a) the food does not, on the basis of the scientific evidence available, pose a safety risk to human health; (b) the food's intended use does not mislead the consumer, especially when the food is intended to replace another food and there is a significant change in the nutritional value; (c) where the food is intended to replace another food, it does not differ from that food in such a way that its normal consumption would be nutritionally disadvantageous for the consumer.

The procedure for placing novel foods on the EU market is described under Article 10 of the Regulation. Therefore, the conditions under which a novel food may be marketed are laid down at European level and are designed to ensure maximum protection for consumers.

At present, based on the aforementioned Novel Foods Regulation, the marketing of cultured meat is not permitted due to the absence of prior authorization. The two applications submitted to date (one in July 2024 and one in January 2025) to the European Commission are still in the early stages of the authorization process, which will involve the Commission, the European Food Safety Authority (EFSA) and the Standing

Committee on Plants, Animals, Food and Feed (PAFF Committee) (Volpato, 2022).

Cultured meat is sometimes perceived as a challenge, particularly by farmers and meat professionals, whose sector has already been weakened. This concern goes even further, with fears about the future of our countryside, particularly in terms of maintaining the landscape and rural activity.

But the European debate on cultivated meat did not begin with these submissions. In recent years, EFSA has promoted scientific experiments on cell-based alternative foods with the aim of stimulating discussion among experts and identifying possible scenarios. The controversial nature of the subject matter and the political pressure arising from the significant underlying interests have prompted some national legislators to adopt national regulations on lab-grown products that are restrictive or totally prohibitive.

For instance, in December 2023, the Italian legislator approved Law No. 172 of 1 December 2023, "Provisions on the prohibition of the production and placing on the market of food and feed consisting of, isolated from or produced from cell cultures or tissues derived from vertebrate animals, as well as the prohibition of the designation of meat for processed products containing vegetable proteins".

In particular, the objectives of the law are clearly set out in Article 1, which states that the law aims to «ensure the protection of human health and the interests of citizens», as well as to «preserve the agri-food heritage, as a set of products that reflect Italy's socio-economic and cultural evolution and are of strategic importance to the national interest». The provision explicitly states the so-called «imperative requirements of general interest» that justify it: food safety, the protection of consumer interests and the preservation of the social structure linked to agriculture (animal husbandry, related traditional supply chains and products that express national cultural identity). As far as we are concerned here, cultivated meat is subject to a general ban on production, sale and administration (see Article 2) based on the precautionary principle. The ban appears particularly broad, as it covers all stages of the production chain, regardless of whether the product is intended for the Italian or foreign market (see the ban on "producing for export"). With regard to scientific research, some believe that the wording does not seem to prohibit experimentation and research, as the ban on possession is limited to commercial purposes ("possession for sale") or administration, while others believe that it is inevitable and entirely clear that the current legislation (Article 2), by imposing an absolute ban not only on marketing but also on production (it should be reiterated that this prohibition on production applies regardless of subsequent marketing in Italy and, indeed, the law expressly refers to the prohibition on production for export), causes clear and total damage to scientific research, discouraging its funding and limiting the possibilities for experimentation. The latter point of view considers the ban in open contrast with both Article 9, paragraph 1 of the Italian Constitution (according to which «The Republic promotes the development of culture and scientific and technical research») and with European principles, which identify freedom of scientific research as a fundamental right and, at the same time, a tool for scientific and social progress and sustainability, also taking into account that freedom of scientific research implies the right to collect and process empirical materials (see, among many other sources, Article 13 of the Charter of Fundamental Rights of the European Union and the Motion for a resolution with recommendations to the Commission on promoting scientific research freedom in the EU Resolution 2023/2184). Therefore, the resulting risk is that the entire research sector in Italy will find no way to progress or contribute to the supranational scientific debate on these issues, in open contrast to the very purpose of protecting human health, which presupposes the vitality of scientific research (Cerini, 2025).

However, beyond the criticisms that have been levelled at the law in question, both from a procedural point of view (since it was adopted in violation of the rules on prior TRIS notification before the adoption of the measure) and from a content point of view, especially for the improper reference to the precautionary principle, these considerations aim to highlight the link between Italian culture and culinary tradition that motivated the ban in question to protect the so-called Made in Italy.

3 The Protection of Traditional Food Products in Italy

In order to understand the role played by traditional food products in Italy, it is worth examining some regulatory measures that offer broad protection and significant recognition to such products.

In particular, Ministerial Decree No. 350 of 8 September 1997 defines traditional agri-food products as those products whose processing, preservation and maturing procedures have become deeply rooted over time. Article 2 of the aforementioned decree establishes that each Region is required to draw up its own list of traditional agri-food products, while the Ministry of Agriculture must draw up a national list of all products identified by the Regions and autonomous provinces. The list is periodically updated and supplemented (the latest version dates back to 19 March 2025).

One of the richest categories on the list of traditional food products is fresh and cooked meat. For each product, the Ministerial Decree requires the following information to be provided: the name, characteristics, processing methods, preservation and ageing methods established over time based on local customs. Other important information includes the specific materials and equipment used for the preparation, conditioning or packaging of the products, description of the processing, storage and maturing premises.

Among the most distinctive aspects of the regulation there is the general exception formulated under Article 4 of the Decree about the food hygiene provisions laid down in Community law. Obviously, this exception is applicable on condition that consumers are guaranteed a satisfactory level of hygiene and disinfection of the materials in contact with the product and the premises where production activities are carried out, safeguarding the typical characteristics, healthiness and safety of the product. The regulatory reference for this exception at European level can be found in Commission Regulation (EC) No 2074/2005 of 5 December 2005 laying down implementing measures for certain products, which in Article 7 provides for a derogation from Regulation (EC) No 852/2004 and lays down specific provisions for "food products with traditional characteristics". The scope of the derogation is closely linked to the national law of the Member States: such products must be:

> (a) recognised historically as traditional products, or (b) manufactured according to codified or registered technical references to the traditional process, or according to traditional production methods, or (c) protected as traditional food products by a Community, national, regional or local law.

For "food products with traditional characteristics", Member States may grant individual or general derogations to establishments that are manufacturing them (Paoloni & Barbarossa, 2025).

Additionally, Law No. 172/2023 emphasizes this deep connection between national culture and culinary tradition in the preparatory work report:

> Article 1 of the bill sets out the aims of the measure, containing provisions aimed at ensuring the protection of human health and the interests of citizens, as well as preserving the agri-food heritage, as a set of products that are an expression of Italy's socio-economic and cultural evolution. The value of this process is recognised as being of strategic importance for national interest (paragraph 1). Italy's agri-food heritage is therefore one of our Country's strengths; it consists of highly competitive products that meet expectations in terms of authenticity and reputation, reaching a wide variety of international markets and enjoying excellent commercial success. As specified in the provision in question, it has therefore taken on social and cultural as well as economic significance. Support for agri-food products, traditions and practices is recognised internationally by UNESCO in the context of the protection of the intangible heritage of humanity under the Convention for the Safeguarding of the Intangible Heritage concluded in Paris on 17 October 2003 and ratified by Law No. 167 of 27 September 2007.

In particular, Article 1 of the Convention provides, among its objectives, for the safeguarding of intangible cultural heritage and respect for the intangible cultural heritage of the communities, groups and individuals concerned. Article 2 contains the definition of «intangible cultural heritage» as the set of practices, representations, expressions, knowledge and know-how that communities recognize as part of their cultural heritage. This intangible cultural heritage, according to the same provision, is constantly recreated by communities in response to their environment and history, giving them a sense of identity and continuity. Article 16 of the same Convention sets forth that the Intergovernmental Committee for the Safeguarding of Intangible Cultural Heritage (one of the bodies established by the Convention pursuant to Article 5) shall establish a representative list of the intangible heritage of humanity in order to ensure greater visibility of intangible cultural heritage, raise awareness of its significance and encourage dialogue that respects cultural diversity. Pursuant to Article 12 of the aforementioned Convention, each State is required to draw up one or more inventories in order to safeguard its intangible cultural heritage.

Italian Ministerial Decree No. 3424 of 2017 has then established the National Inventory of Italian Agri-food Heritage (in Italian "INPAI") at the current Ministry of Agriculture, Food Sovereignty and Forestry with the aim of «identifying, cataloguing and documenting cultural elements related to typical Italian agri-food traditions». The Decree defines "agri-food cultural element" as the set of practices, representations, expressions and knowledge relating to food and nutrition culture whose persistence has been documented for at least twenty years, and which communities recognize as part of their intangible agri-food cultural heritage. It also describes the procedure for inclusion in the inventory, as well as the procedure for identifying the "Agri-food Heritage of the Year", i.e., the agri-food cultural element designated as particularly representative and emblematic of the rural and agri-food context and the intangible cultural heritage associated with it. In this regard, it should be noted that Italy holds the world record for UNESCO recognitions in the agri-food sector, having obtained five such recognitions.

In addition, the 2021 "legge di bilancio" (Law 178/2020: Article 1, paragraph 582) provided for the establishment, by Ministerial Decree, the National Observatory for UNESCO Intangible Heritage, which is tasked with identifying the Country's intangible assets and disseminating knowledge about them, promoting research and data collection in this regard and fostering relations with local and international bodies, supporting the development of intercultural dialogue, taking into account the essential link between intangible cultural heritage, tangible cultural heritage and natural assets. The preservation of Italy's agri-food heritage is pursued through the protection of the quality of agri-food products, which is one of Italy's main (agri-food) policy objectives, given that Italy has the highest number of registered trademark products, which are subject to numerous attempts at counterfeiting. In this sense, at the national level, to protect the quality and authenticity of the product itself, the Italian legislator has always reserved great importance to the possibility of mandatorily indicating the national origin of agri-food production. Law No. 4 of 3 February 2011, containing "Provisions on the labelling and quality of food products", laid down the obligation in Articles 4 and 5 for food products marketed, processed, partially processed or unprocessed, to also indicate the place of origin or provenance on the label.

Italy's agri-food heritage has been the subject of recent legislative measures aimed at protecting it, like the Food Sovereignty Fund, with a budget of €25 million for each of the years 2023–2026. The purpose is to promote and support excellence in Italian catering and pastry-making, to enhance the value of Italy's agri-food and wine and food heritage, including through measures to encourage the promotion of products with designation of origin and geographical indication and Italian agri-food excellence, investments in professional equipment and other durable capital goods, as well as measures to support young graduates in the food and wine and hotel hospitality sectors.

4 Possible Scenarios

At present, cultured meat stands at a decisive juncture with multiple potential pathways: the first path foresees the collapse of the cultured meat sector, caused by start-ups unable to meet expectations, insufficient institutional backing, and consumers who continue to doubt its value. In such a case, the market for alternative proteins could either expand or contract. This option reflects a technocratic stagnation scenario, mainly influenced by the perception of risks and the resistance of both stakeholders and consumers to adopt cultured meat.

The second path is the opposite: a future supported by substantial financial resources, remarkable scientific progress, and encouragement from governments and buyers, resulting in a drastic reduction of industrial livestock farming, progressively substituted with cultured meat. This would also require a drastic fall in production expenses. Under such conditions, pragmatic buyers would embrace it above all for its affordability. Within this context, only extensive, positively regarded livestock production would endure, intended to provide a type of meat considered a luxury product. This corresponds to a rapid advancement scenario. It would be sustained by innovation, strong consumer acceptance, and widespread diffusion of cultured meat, generating profound and lasting transformations in food systems.

The third path represents an intermediate position: traditional livestock farming would remain widespread among consumers strongly tied to meat and their culinary identities, while substitutes, including cultured meat, would gain ground mostly for environmental and ethical reasons. Hybrid solutions, blending plant-based proteins with cultured meat, would likely appear first, given the still elevated costs of cultivated muscle tissue. Yet, the limited distribution of cultured meat alone would represent a significant barrier to resolving current ethical and ecological issues. This outlook corresponds to a promising circumstances scenario, marked by a favourable cultural climate towards cultured meat and a gradual incorporation of this product as an additional option available on the market (Moritz et al., 2023).

Currently, the real situation is closer to path 1, since cultured meat is still absent from the mainstream market. Its commercialization has so far been authorized in Singapore, in the United States and Israel. Path 2 seems the least plausible, given the numerous technical, legal, cultural and social obstacles still present. The unresolved question is whether a shift towards path 3 is possible, which remains uncertain due to the many regulatory, political, scientific and, as in the case discussed in this article, cultural barriers, due to the strong connections between culinary traditions and national identity (Hoquette et al., 2025).

5 Conclusions

The issues involved concern not only the protection of human health, consumer information and the free movement of food products within a common market, but also broader issues, or rather issues that cut across individual fields of disciplinary investigation, such as the environment and the climate crisis, which in themselves fuel the search for technological innovations capable of curbing the unsustainable effects of food consumption.

There is a clear need for lawyers and policymakers to engage in vigorous interdisciplinary dialogue, not least in order to avoid undermining the Sustainable Development Goals (SDGs), which widely reveal the need to move beyond anthropological perspective on law. Indeed, it is well known that the twenty-first century has brought with it a renewed legal dogma, which unites people, the environment and animals through the filter of an idea of sustainability that can be interpreted from multiple perspectives. With specific reference to the use of meat, there is a widely recognized global desire to promote more moderate consumption in order to reduce the carbon footprint of livestock farming through various means, including technological innovation.

It is also important to adopt legal and political frameworks for cultivated meat that take into account the evidence underlying the One Health concept (see Russo Corvace G. chapter in this Volume), i.e., the recognition that the health of humans, domestic and wild animals, plants and the environment in general (including ecosystems) is closely linked and interdependent (v. joint tripartite (FAO, OIE, WHO) and UnEP Statement—OHHLEP's definition of "One Health"). In fact, the One Health Approach refers to the collaborative effort between different disciplines aimed at achieving an optimal level of health for humans (human health), animals (animal health) and the environment (environmental health).

The translation of the One Health paradigm into regulatory choices and policies is by no means free from critical issues and limitations, but at the same time, there is no doubt that this concept can be fruitfully implemented in the areas of food safety and technological innovation. In this context, in addition to an important prescriptive content (i.e., the indication that an adequate level of food safety for humans cannot be achieved without the production, distribution and consumption of food being carried out with respect for animal health and environmental protection), the One-Health paradigm also indicates a precise method: the use of regulatory choices that are the result of a holistic and multidisciplinary approach (Lanni & Ragone, 2025). This means that regulatory options relating to food and, even more so, to novel foods must be taken within decision-making processes in which all relevant expertise is considered (as far as possible). Not only that: the literature has highlighted that full implementation of the paradigm «will not be achieved without a philosophical shift from the expert-controlled, top-down paradigm that still dominates both science and medicine [... to ...] a broader, more democratic approach» (Karesh & Cook, 2005). In this sense, the One-Health concept does not seem far removed from the application of the instruments of deliberative democracy mentioned above.

The Italian case discussed is a paradigmatic example of how cultural and social interests anchored in culinary tradition can prevail over the potential environmental benefits of producing and consuming cultivated meat, even though the data are still too limited. One of the aims of this paper was to demonstrate the multiplicity of aspects and interests that come to the fore in attempts to advance food biotechnologies in the context of sustainable development. In fact, to date, the Green Deal and, in particular, the From Farm to Fork strategy have achieved limited results, exclusively in areas where they do not involve a radical and substantial change in food systems, as in the case of the regulation of new genomic techniques, on which there is no harmonization between the legislators of the various Member States.

What is certain is that in the complex dialogue between law and science, legislators should avoid any extreme and ideological positions, such as, on the one hand, supporting and applying technological progress at all costs and, on the other, adhering to irrational fears of innovation and believing that the new is necessarily the enemy of tradition.

Consequently, a comprehensive risk assessment of all the factors at play, conducted by independent experts, appears crucial. An integrated and systematic scientific approach must consider not only studies relating to human health profiles, but also environmental, socio-economic and cultural considerations. The broad debate on new technologies, and on cultured meat, must be reconsidered considering this complex context.

In any case, it is almost impossible to predict the future scenario for cultured meat due to the lack of sufficient scientific data and the presence of significant critical issues and obstacles to its dissemination. European policymakers need to initiate a constructive debate with member Countries to ensure a shared legal and political response to technological innovations.

References

Albisinni, F. (2025). Quale carne? In *Quaderni della rivista di diritto alimentare*, 1 (pp. 104–112).

Albisinni, F., & Costato, L. (2023). *Trattato breve di diritto agrario italiano e dell'Unione Europea* (4th ed.). Cedam.

Benozzo, M. (2012). La disciplina delle biotecnologie tra scelte di politica comune e sviluppo territoriale. *Agricoltura istituzioni mercati, 1*, 55–68.

Benozzo, M. (2018). *Biotecnologie agroalimentari. Profili di tutela e responsabilità*. Aracne.

Benozzo, M. (2023). *Biotecnologie alimentari e nuove tecniche di miglioramento genetico tra Unione Europea e Stati Uniti*. Aracne.

Bruno, F. (2000a). Il principio di precauzione tra diritto dell'Unione Europea e WTO. *Dir. e giur. agr. e ambiente*, 569.

Bruno, F. (2000b). Principio di precauzione e organismi geneticamente modificati. In *Dir. e giur. agr. e ambiente*, II.

Bruno, F. (2017). *Il diritto alimentare nel contesto globale: USA e UE a confronto.* Cedam.

Bruno, F. (2022). *Il diritto alimentare. Sviluppo sostenibile e tutela della salute.* Cedam.

Bryant, C. J., & Barnett, J. C. (2019). What's in a name? Consumer perceptions of in vitro meat under different names. *Appetite, 137*, 104–113. https://doi.org/10.1016/j.appet.2019.02.021

Castellani, P., Cassia, F., Vargas-Sánchez, A., & Giaretta, E. (2025). Food innovation towards a sustainable world: A study on intention to purchase lab-grown meat. *Technological Forecasting & Social Change*, 211. https://doi.org/10.1016/j.techfore.2024.123912

Cerini, D. (2025). "From farm to fork" vs. "From factory to lab": riflessioni su sostenibilità sociale e benessere animale a partire dalla l.172/2023. *Quaderni della rivista di diritto alimentare, 1*, 76–103.

Chodkowska, K. A., Wodz, K., & Wojciechowski, J. (2022). Sustainable future protein foods: The challenges and the future of cultivated meat. *Foods, 11*, 4008. https://doi.org/10.3390/foods11244008

Choudhury, D., Tseng, T. W., & Swartz, E. (2020). The business of cultured meat. *Trends in Biotechnology, 38*(6), 573–577. https://doi.org/10.1016/j.tibtech.2020.02.012

Chriki, S., & Hocquette, J.-F. (2020). The myth of cultured meat: A review. *Frontiers in Nutrition., 7*, 7. https://doi.org/10.3389/fnut.2020.00007

FAO, UNEP, WHO, WOAH. (2023). *A guide to implementing of the one health joint plan of action at national level*. https://openknowledge.fao.org/items/d5be526e-36a6-4c90-8b7c-75ac01bc340c

FAO, WHO. (2023). *Food safety aspects of cell-based food*. https://doi.org/10.4060/cc4855en

Formici, G., "Meating" the future: alcune riflessioni sulla necessità di promuovere un attento dibattito regolatorio in materia di c.d. carne sintetica. *Forum di Quaderni Costituzionali*, II/2023, 16.

Germanò, A. (2022). *Manuale di diritto agrario* (9th ed.). G. Giappichelli.

Holle, M. (2025). Sustainability in European agri-food law. In L. Costato, F. Albisinni, & T. Georgopoulos (Eds.), *European and Global Food Law* (pp. 409–419). Cedam.

Hoquette, J.-F., Chriki, S., Fournier, D., & Ellies-Oury, M.-P. (2025). Review: Will "cultured meat" transform our food system towards more sustainability? *Animal, 19*(Suppl 1), 101145. https://doi.org/10.1016/j.animal.2024.101145

Jetzke, T. et al. (2022). *Meat of the future: Trend report for assessing the environmental impacts of plant-based substitutes, edible insects, and in vitro meat*. www.umweltbundesamt.de/publikationen.

Karesh, W. B., & Cook, R. A. (2005). The human-animal link. *Foreign Affairs, 4*(2005), 50.

Lanni, S., & Ragone, G. (2025). Il rapporto tra novel foods e carne coltivata. *Quaderni della rivista di diritto alimentare, 1*, 17–32.

Lanzoni, D., Rebucci, R., Formici, G., Cheli, F., Ragone, G., Baldi, A., Violini, L., Sundaram, T. S., & Giromini, C. (2024). Cultured meat in the European

Union: Legislative context and food safety issues. *Current Research in Food Science., 16*(8), Article 100722. https://doi.org/10.1016/j.crfs.2024.100722
Lisboa, H. M., et al. (2024). Innovative and sustainable food preservation techniques: Enhancing food quality, safety, and environmental sustainability. *Sustainability, 16*(18). https://doi.org/10.3390/su16188223
Mancini, M. C., & Antonioli, F. (2020). Il ruolo dell'informazione nell'accettazione di novel food da parte del consumatore: il caso della carne coltivata. *BioLaw Journal, 2*(2020), 104–106.
Mancini, M. C., & Antonioli, F. (2022a). The future of cultured meat between sustainability expectations and socio-economic challenges. In R. Bhat (Eds.), *Future foods: Global trends, opportunities, and sustainability challenges* (pp. 331–350). Academic Press.
Mancini, M. C., & Antonioli, F. (2022b). Italian consumers standing at the crossroads of alternative protein sources: Cultivated meat, insect-based and novel plant-based foods. *Meat Science*. https://doi.org/10.1016/j.meatsci.2022.108942
Moritz, et al. (2023). A multi-level perspective of potential transition pathways towards cultured meat: Finnish and German political stakeholder perceptions. *Research Policy, 52*. https://doi.org/10.1016/j.respol.2023.104866
Nzietchueng, S., Kitua, A., Nyatanyi, T., & Rwego, I. B. (2023). Facilitating implementation of the one health approach: A definition of a one health intervention. *One Health, 16*, Article 100491. https://doi.org/10.1016/j.onehlt.2023.100491
Palmieri, N., Perito, M. A., & Lupi, C. (2020). Consumer acceptance of cultured meat: Some hints from Italy. *British Food Journal, 123*(1), 109–123. https://doi.org/10.1108/BFJ-02-2020-0092
Paoloni, L., & Barbarossa, D. (2025). Traditional food. In L. Costato, F. Albisinni, & T. Georgopoulos (Eds.), *European and global food law* (pp. 672–680). Cedam.
Post, M. J., et al. (2020). Scientific, sustainability and regulatory challenges of cultured meat. *Nature Food, 1*, 403–415. https://doi.org/10.1038/s43016-020-0112-z
Qu, B., Xiao, Z., Upadhyay, A., & Luo, Y. (2024). Perspectives on sustainable food production system: Characteristics and green technologies. *Journal of Agriculture and Food Research, 12*. https://doi.org/10.1016/j.jafr.2024.100988
Ragone, G. (2022). One Health e Costituzione italiana, tra spinte eco-centriche e nuove prospettive di tutela della salute umana, ambientale e animale. One World, One Health… Which law? *Corti supreme e salute, 3*, 809–826.

Rubino, V. (2025). Sustainability in European agri-food law. In L. Costato, F. Albisinni, & T. Georgopoulos (Eds.), *European and global food law* (pp. 893–900). Cedam.

Saija, R. (2025a). Carni e pesci in vitro. Quali regole in vista della sostenibilità? *Quaderni della rivista di diritto alimentare, 1*, 33–44.

Saija, R. (2025b). Food, religion, and ethics. In L. Costato, F. Albisinni, & T. Georgopoulos (Eds.), *European and global food law* (pp. 312–322). Cedam.

Scaffardi, L., & Formici, G. (2025). Cell-based meat. In L. Costato, F. Albisinni, & T. Georgopoulos (Eds.), *European and global food law* (pp. 714–727). Cedam.

Seehafer, A., & Bartles, M. (2019). Meat 2.0—The regulatory environment of plant-based and cultured meat. *European Food and Feed Law Review, 14*, 323–331.

Sekhar, M., Rastogi, M., Rajesh, C. M., Saikanth, D. R. K., Rout, S., Kumar, S., & Amit Kumar, P. (2024). Exploring traditional agricultural techniques integrated with modern farming for a sustainable future: A review. *Journal of Scientific Research and Reports*. https://doi.org/10.9734/jsrr/2024/v30i31871

Shafique, M., Kurshid, M., Muzammil, et al. (2024). Traversed dynamics of climate change and One Health. *Environmental Sciences Europe, 36*, 135. https://doi.org/10.1186/s12302-024-00931-8

Singh, M. (2024). Exploring the intersection of nutrition, gastronomy, and sustainability: A comprehensive review of contemporary food trends, dietary practices, and future directions in culinary health. *International Journal for Multidimensional Research Perspectives, 2*.

Violini, L. (2023). *One health: dal paradigma alle implicazioni giuridiche*. Giappichelli.

Vlčko, T., et al. (2023). Cell-based meat labelling—Current worldwide legislation status. *Annals of Animal Science, 23*, 927–938. https://doi.org/10.2478/aoas-2022-0092

Volpato, A. (2022). Novel foods in the EU integrated administrative space: An institutional perspective. In L. Scaffardi & G. Formici (Eds.), *Novel foods and edible insects in the European Union. An interdisciplinary analysis* (pp. 15–36). Springer.

FSC
www.fsc.org
MIX
Papier | Fördert
gute Waldnutzung
FSC® C083411

Kolibri 360 GmbH
Ferdinand-Jühlke-Straße 7
99095 Erfurt, Deutschland
produktsicherheit@kolibri360.de